How I reversed Type 2 Diabetes, healed from severe neuropathy and lost 41 lbs in 6 months

By Brian Babayans

Introduction

In 2010, I was diagnosed with Type 2 Diabetes. Like most people I didn't even know I had it. I didn't have any symptoms until it was too late. When I realized something was wrong and I was constantly fatigued and couldn't lose weight no matter how much I exercised or dieted, I went to the doctor and requested a full set of labs to be performed to find out what was happening to me. When the blood test showed an elevated glucose level, I had further tests performed to confirm that the results of my Hemoglobin A1c had gone up to 6.8, which is full-blown diabetes. A few months later, I developed severe neuropathy and could barely walk. My hands, feet, legs, and toes were completely numb and I couldn't even walk up a flight of stairs. I also began to develop a cataract in one eye and my vision was becoming blurry. I went to numerous doctors and specialty clinics that offered treatment for diabetes and neuropathy. In a matter of 6 months I had completely reversed my diabetes, lost 41 pounds, completely healed from neuropathy, and was in better shape than I had been in 15 years.

For the majority of my life I had been involved in sports, athletic activities, and/or weight training. It wasn't until I began to have severe allergy problems due to the Santa Ana winds in Southern California that I was unable to work out the way I used to. My blood sugar rose due to bad diet and lack of exercise.

While I was going through this nightmare, I tried to find one book or video that explained everything about the condition and how to reverse it. Unfortunately, there wasn't one particular resource to be found. Every medical professional I spoke with said that diabetes could be reversed through diet and exercise but none of them gave me detailed comprehensive information in order to do so. Over time, I did find the answers, but they were scattered and varied, requiring a lot of time, energy, and testing of different diet plans, exercises, and research on my own body for me to put proven solutions together myself in one all-inclusive book - this one. I went to a holistic facility in Newport Beach, CA and met with doctors who specialized in Type 2 diabetes and learned of alternative and natural ways to reverse diabetes and heal from neuropathy. I watched numerous videos and researched numerous websites and read several books all to learn how to successfully heal myself naturally from diabetes.

This book is that one resource I wish was available when I needed it most. I'm sharing my story and the things I learned in one place so that you won't have to search for information like I did. I provide information to some treatment facilities that offer alternative therapies, remedies, and supplements.

I go into the details of my diet during this time and explain exactly what I ate. I want to provide you with the right tools so that you can make a full recovery as well - not only from diabetes, from excessive weight gain, low energy, costly and painful surgeries, reliance on medications with bad side effects and diminished lifespan. Most importantly, I have blood tests, Body Mass Index tests, and before and after pictures as proof that the claims I'm making in this book are real.

This book can help you save money instead of spending it on doctors, hospitals, and medications to fight disease. It also serves as a preventative measure against getting diabetes in the first place, and as such, this information is not just limited to diabetics. It was written for anyone who wants to have a healthy lifestyle, stay in shape, eat right, and fuel their body correctly to give it the energy it needs. If you follow the methods within this book and apply them to your life, your chances of developing diabetes, heart disease, high blood pressure, neuropathy, cancer, and other life-threatening illnesses will decrease - and your *quality of life* will increase instead. You will lose weight and also lose the food addictions that are caused by the Standard American Diet that is filled with processed chemicals and sugars.

Another reason I wrote this book is because during my research of medicines for neuropathy, I learned that one of the medications can lead to suicidal thoughts and some of the people who have used it actually have committed suicide, including children. When I learned this, I couldn't sleep at night. I knew I had to share all the knowledge I learned with the world and if I can save one life with this book I will have accomplished my goal.

Diabetes is becoming an epidemic in the world, especially the United States, and more people need this information than ever before. The good news is that diabetes is completely reversible through diet, exercise, and supplementation. It is truly amazing how quickly the body adapts and changes to a proper diet and exercise. The human body is a non-stop healing machine. It was designed to be self-repairing and self-healing.

In this book you'll learn:

- What Type 2 diabetes is and the dangers associated with this condition
- How to find out if you have Type 2 Diabetes or elevated blood sugar in 10 minutes
- How to reverse your blood sugar levels using diet, exercise, and supplementation
- The healthiest foods to eat (as well as what not to eat)
- The best way to eat to stabilize your blood sugar levels (including portion sizes and fasting)
- Which supplements to take and how they will support your healing (especially from symptoms like neuropathy)
- The best exercise program to burn glucose quickly and keep it low. (I also include a complete full body exercise program, which I have used for the past 25 years)
- Information on alternative treatments and facilities that specialize in reversing and healing from diabetes. These facilities have specialized treatments for advanced stages of Type 2 diabetes to prevent amputations, heal neuropathy, and reverse the condition
- Blood tests showing my blood sugar levels before, during, and after my treatment along with Body Mass Index results showing the progress of lean muscle mass and weight loss.
- Additional healing treatments for detoxifying the liver, increasing your immune system, and improving your overall health
- Before and after pictures showing the dramatic change in my overall appearance

*Note: Please talk to your doctor before following the program outlined in this book. I am not a licensed medical doctor, nurse, or physician's assistant. I do not have a degree in medicine, nor am I licensed to practice medicine in any state or country. This book is a compilation of the things that I learned and applied in order to heal myself from Type 2 Diabetes and severe neuropathy. It is intended to be an educational resource that can be shared with your doctor in order to decide which form of treatment is best for you.

Table of Contents

Chapter One

How To Find Out If You Have Type 2 Diabetes Right Now

A1C Home testing kit

The fastest way to see if you have diabetes or elevated blood sugar is to take the Hemoglobin A1C test. This test measures your blood sugar during the last 2-3 months. You can determine what your blood sugar levels are within ten minutes by purchasing A1C System home testing kit. They can be found at most major drugstores or online and cost approximately $25.

If you're diagnosed with A1C levels above 6.3, you technically have Type 2 diabetes. Your doctor will probably recommend that you buy a daily glucose monitoring meter. You will also need to purchase some of the blood measuring strips, which are sold separately and with a prescription. Most blood test monitoring kits save the results for up to three months with hundreds of measurements and can also give you a 7-day, 14-day, and 30 day average. However, I still highly recommend getting an A1C test, which will accurately give you the results of a 2-3 month period.

Chapter Two

What Is Type 2 Diabetes?

Medical terms related to Diabetes and health symptoms associated with it

Without going into much detail, I am going to explain most of the important medical terminology associated with diabetes and related health issues. It is important to understand this terminology since it will be used by your physicians throughout your treatment.

Definition of diabetes

The origin of word diabetes comes from the Greeks, and it means "siphon" which is a symptom of frequent urination one suffers when they have the disease. "Diabetes" is also referred to as diabetes mellitus – literally meaning "siphon honey", alluding to the sugar found in the urine of diabetics.

Type 2 Diabetes is caused when your blood glucose (blood sugar) levels are too high over a long period of time, causing damage to your internal organs and body. Glucose comes from the foods you eat - mostly carbohydrates and sugar. The body stores energy in two ways - as sugar and as fat. Normally, the hormone insulin is released by the pancreas to help glucose get absorbed into your cells and used as energy. If the sugar in your body doesn't get used as energy, it gets stored as fat. Over time, if all of the energy storage in your body has been exhausted, sugar spills into the bloodstream and your glucose levels become high. When this happens insulin is unable to work properly to get energy into the cells through sugar. This is what's known as "insulin resistance" and is the root cause of diabetic problems.

In Type 2 Diabetes, the body does not use insulin well. Blood sugar doesn't get absorbed, or there isn't enough insulin available and the glucose remains in the blood. This excess glucose in your body is the main cause for damage to your kidneys, nerves, and eyes, and can also lead to heart disease, stroke, and hardening of the arteries.

Pre-diabetes

Pre-diabetes occurs when your blood sugar levels are between 5.7 and 6.3 and is measured by the Hemoglobin A1c test. Any A1C level between 5.7 and 6.4 percent is considered pre-diabetic. Anything above 6.3 percent is considered full blown diabetes. Normal glucose levels are anywhere from 4.0 to 5.6.

Insulin Resistance

Insulin resistance occurs when your cells are no longer able to absorb glucose, causing them to become "resistant" to insulin, the hormone that's responsible for helping your cells absorb sugars for energy. Insulin enters cells first by binding to target insulin receptors. Diabetics (and some people who have pre-diabetes) have impaired glucose tolerance. In these individuals, blood glucose rises to abnormally high levels. This may be due to a lack of insulin released by the pancreas or a failure of target cells and tissues to respond to the insulin present in the body (or both), causing insulin resistance and eventually, damage to your nerves and organs.

Metabolic Syndrome (also known as Syndrome X)

Metabolic syndrome means basically that your metabolism isn't metabolizing nutrients and energy properly. It is a term used to describe if you have 3 out of 5 of the following medical conditions:

- Abdominal obesity
- Elevated blood pressure
- Elevated fasting glucose or A1c levels
- High triglycerides, High density cholesterol (LDL) and low high-density cholesterol (HDL) levels
- Fatty liver

Ketones

Ketone is a chemical produced when there is a shortage of insulin in the blood and the body breaks down body fat for energy. Ketones in the urine is a sign that your body is using fat for energy instead of using glucose because not enough insulin is available to use glucose for energy.

Ketones build up in the blood and urine as fats and are broken down for energy. In high levels, ketones can be very dangerous and even poisonous. This serious condition is known as ketoacidosis and, if left untreated, can lead to diabetic coma or even death. The symptoms of ketoacidosis can be confused with others (such as the flu or a stomach virus), so be sure to talk to your doctor about a plan for when to test for ketones.

Fasting Glucose Test

This is the measurement of blood sugar after fasting (not eating any food) for 8 or more hours. Normally, the best time to perform this reading is first thing in the morning before any meals. This gives you the most accurate fasting glucose result. The normal range for this test is 70-100. Anything above 100 is considered out of range.

I would test myself every day in the morning before meals and continue to test it after eating certain meals, as I was experimenting with my diet to determine which foods would keep my glucose levels low.

Glucose Tolerance Test

This test is to determine insulin resistance and is performed in a lab if you've fasted the night before. You will be given three blood tests after drinking a sugary beverage every two hours. Your blood sugar is then tested after each drink. The results will show whether you are insulin resistant and/or diabetic.

I had to take this test myself because I had a very bad reaction to eating sugary foods after following a restricted diet given to me by one of my doctors. The diet consisted of low calorie meals, but still contained sugar and carbohydrates. My doctor's goal was to restrict my diet and the only way he could do that was to give me food that contained a specific number of calories. This included snacks that contained sugars and carborhydrates but were on the healthy end of the spectrum. He didn't know how insulin resistant I was or how bad my diabetes was at the time. When I told him about my reactions to eating his food, he told me to stop immediately. I then designed my own food plan based on what I learned and it is included here in this book.

Cholesterol

Cholesterol is a waxy, fat-like substance that's found in all cells of the body. Your body needs some cholesterol to make hormones, vitamin D, and substances that help you digest foods. Your body makes all the cholesterol it needs. However, cholesterol is also found in some of the foods you eat.

Cholesterol travels through your bloodstream in small packages called lipoproteins. These packages are made of fat (lipids) on the inside and proteins on the outside.

Two kinds of lipoproteins carry cholesterol throughout your body: low-density lipoproteins (LDL) and high-density lipoproteins (HDL). It's important to have healthy levels of both types of lipoproteins. LDL cholesterol sometimes is called "bad" cholesterol. A high LDL level leads to a buildup of cholesterol in your arteries. HDL cholesterol sometimes is called "good" cholesterol. This is because it carries cholesterol from other parts of your body back to your liver. Your liver removes the cholesterol from your body.

High Cholesterol

High blood cholesterol is a condition that usually has no signs or symptoms and many people don't know that their cholesterol levels are too high unless they request a lipid panel blood test from their doctor. The higher the level of LDL cholesterol in your blood, the greater your chance of getting heart disease. The higher the level of HDL cholesterol in your blood, the lower your chance is of getting heart disease.

Coronary heart disease is a condition in which plaque builds up inside the coronary arteries. Plaque is made up of cholesterol, fat, calcium, and other substances found in the blood. When plaque builds up in the arteries, the condition is called atherosclerosis.

Over time, plaque hardens and narrows your coronary arteries. This limits the flow of oxygen-rich blood to the heart. Eventually, an area of plaque can rupture. This causes a blood clot to form on the surface of the plaque. If the clot becomes large enough, it can partially or completely block blood flow through a coronary artery.

If the flow of oxygen-rich blood to your heart muscle is reduced or blocked, it may lead to angina (chest pain) or even heart attack. The pain from angina may also occur in your shoulders, arms, neck, jaw, or back. If blood flow isn't restored quickly, the section of heart muscle begins to die.

Plaque can also build up in other arteries in your body, such as those that bring oxygen-rich blood to your brain and limbs.

Triglycerides

Triglycerides are a type of blood fat. High triglyceride levels are indicative of excess sugar and too much fat in the diet. The excess sugar is combined with the fat and typically stored around the stomach area and around muscles.

Factors that can raise your triglyceride level include

- Being overweight
- Lack of physical activity
- Smoking
- Excessive alcohol use
- A very high carbohydrate diet
- Certain diseases and medicines
- Some genetic disorders

You may be able to lower your triglycerides by taking fish oil supplements, controlling your diet, and exercising. Some foods raise your triglycerides including sugary foods and foods high in saturated fat like cheese, whole milk, and red meat.

When your doctor requests a "lipid profile" blood test, the results will display the HDL, LDL, and triglycerides and include ratios of good to bad cholesterol (see lab results for examples of my lipid profile results).

Chapter Three

Symptoms Of Diabetes, Organ Damage, And Other Complications

Because Type 2 Diabetes can take a long time to develop, you may have the disease and not be aware of it. It may even take years before you experience symptoms. High blood sugar may cause a spike in blood pressure, which can lead to stroke, heart attack, or kidney failure. It's important to know the signs, so I've included them below. These are the first symptoms you will most likely experience if you've become diabetic.

Symptoms of Type 2 Diabetes

- Increased thirst
- Increased urination
- Lower Back pain
- Increased hunger (especially after eating)
- Dry mouth
- Nausea and sometimes vomiting
- Fatigue
- Blurred vision
- Numbness or tingling of the hands and feet (also known as neuropathy)

- Frequent infections of the skin, urinary tract, or vagina
- Sores which are slow to heal
- Dizziness when standing up (caused by neuropathy)

Complications Associated With Type 2 Diabetes

If Type 2 Diabetes isn't under control, a number of serious or life-threatening complications may arise. Here is a short summary of the issues that may occur over time and will be explained in further detail:

- **Retinopathy and/or blurred vision:** Vision gets worse over time as diabetes progresses.
- **Kidney damage:** Over time, your kidneys may become damaged due to excess blood sugar and/or high blood pressure and may eventually fail, leading to the need to receive a transplant or be put on dialysis. Dialysis is a treatment which replaces the functions of the kidneys, which involves using a device to cleanse your blood.
- **High blood pressure:** This occurs especially after eating meals with high sugar content or those that are high on the glycemic index (foods which convert to sugar quickly in the body). This can also lead to heart palpitations
- **Neuropathy (poor blood circulation and nerve damage):** Damage to the blood vessels can lead to a higher risk of stroke and heart attack as well as peripheral artery disease. Damage to nerves and hardening of arteries leads to a decline of physical sensation, as well as poor blood circulation in the feet. This condition eventually increases the chances of

receiving infections and skin ulcers, creating a high risk for amputation. Damage to nerves may also lead to digestive problems, such as nausea, vomiting, and diarrhea.

- **Heart attack or stroke:** High blood pressure caused by spikes in glucose can lead to stroke or heart attack.
- **Atherosclerosis** – As explained earlier, plaque may begin to build up in the arteries due to elevated levels of cholesterol and high triglycerides. Over time, the plaque hardens and narrows the arteries. Eventually, an area of plaque can rupture. When this happens, blood cell fragments called platelets stick to the site of the injury. They may clump together to form blood clots. Clots narrow the arteries even more, limiting the flow of oxygen-rich blood to your body.

Retinopathy

In Type 2 Diabetes, retinopathy occurs when high blood sugar levels damage the tiny vessels in the eye, causing them to leak blood and other fluids. When this happens, the retinal tissue swells and vision becomes cloudy or blurry. This can eventually lead to separation of the retina, cataracts and even blindness. Reducing your blood sugar levels and cholesterol levels will enable your eyesight to return to normal, like mine did. I had blurry vision for a few months when my blood sugar was really high, but when my body completely healed, my vision improved dramatically. I also began to develop cataracts, which eventually healed after I recovered from neuropathy.

Kidney Damage

Diabetes is the most common cause of kidney failure. Since high blood sugar damages the small vessels in the body, it affects the ones in your kidneys as well, harming the nephrons within that are responsible for filtering waste products and other toxins from your body. When this occurs, the kidneys also lose some of the other important functions your body needs such as excreting urea and ammonium, preventing high blood pressure, and/or producing necessary hormones and enzymes. Many of the symptoms like fatigue, nausea, and vomiting listed on the previous page, are indications that your kidneys are being affected by diabetes.

One of the earliest signs of kidney problems is that there is leakage of albumin into the urine. This can only be detected by a urine test. Albumin is a protein that's heavily involved in transporting molecules throughout the body, as well as binding with toxins so that they can be removed before they can be absorbed within the organs and tissues.

If your disease persists over an extended period of time, you may need to receive dialysis treatment or have a kidney transplant.

Dialysis Treatment

When your kidneys fail, dialysis keeps your body in balance by:

- removing waste, salt, and extra water to prevent them from building up in the body

- keeping a safe level of certain chemicals in your blood, such as potassium, sodium, and bicarbonate
- helping to control blood pressure

There are two types of dialysis - hemodialysis and peritoneal dialysis.

In hemodialysis, an artificial kidney (hemodialyzer) is used to remove waste and extra chemicals and fluid from your blood. To get your blood into the artificial kidney, the doctor needs to make an entrance into your blood vessels. This is done by making a small incision in your arm or leg. However, if your blood vessels are not adequate for a fistula, the doctor may use a soft plastic tube to join an artery and a vein under your skin. This is called a graft.

Occasionally, an access is made by means of a narrow plastic tube, called a catheter, which is inserted into a large vein in your neck. This type of access may be temporary, but is sometimes used for long-term treatment.

Kidney failure is usually permanent but not always. Some kinds of acute kidney failure get better after treatment. In some cases of acute kidney failure, dialysis may only be needed for a short time until the kidneys get better. In chronic or end-stage kidney failure, your kidneys do not recover and you'll need dialysis for the rest of your life. If your doctor says you're a candidate, you may choose to be placed on a waiting list for a new kidney.

If you do need to have a kidney transplant, you'll have to wait for a donor, and even if you are able to find one, there's no guarantee your body will accept the transplanted kidney. It may reject it no matter how close the match is. It's much better to take care of the one you have.

High Blood Pressure

High blood pressure (or hypertension) is asymptomatic meaning there are no symptoms. Because of this, it's especially important for people with Type 2 Diabetes to be aware of it and do what they can to keep it under control. If left unchecked it can result in stroke, heart attack, kidney failure, aneurisms, or death.

At first, I didn't correlate the spike in my blood sugar to hypertension, but over time I noticed a pattern. As my blood sugar dropped and stayed under 110, my blood pressure also stayed at a normal level. If I ate a high glycemic food loaded with carbohydrates or high fructose corn syrup I noticed that both my blood sugar and blood pressure would spike. This taught me that by keeping my diet clean and eating mostly vegetables and small amounts of animal protein (chicken, salmon, turkey) along with exercise, my blood pressure remains at a normal level.

If you have hypertension or if you're diabetic, you should check your blood pressure at least twice a day (once in the morning when you first wake up and once at night). In the morning you should wait at least 15 minutes after you wake up for a more accurate reading. This is because blood pressure is usually slightly elevated upon first waking since your body is trying to revive itself after hours of inactivity.

The normal range of blood pressure is 120/80. Any reading of 140/90 and higher is considered high blood pressure. The top number (systolic pressure) refers to the amount of pressure in your arteries during contraction of your heart muscle. The bottom number (diastolic pressure) refers to your blood pressure when your heart muscle is between beats.

It is important to note that blood pressure fluctuates throughout the day, especially after physical activity. After any type of physical activity, you should wait at least 15 minutes after to get an accurate reading.

Salt will also affect your blood pressure. The more salt in your food, the higher your blood pressure will be. It is important to reduce your sodium intake as much as possible—especially if you have diabetes because as mentioned earlier, eating a high glycemic meal may spike your blood sugar that will also increase your blood pressure.

It is a very good idea to purchase your own blood pressure monitor. It may save your life. You can buy one at any drug store. I own a wrist monitor that gives a very accurate reading and is comparable to the blood pressure testing device in my doctor's office. On one visit, I brought my wrist monitor into my doctor's office to test the accuracy of the readings, and after they tested my blood pressure with their device I immediately tested my blood pressure on my wrist monitor. The results were only off by a few points in both the systolic and diastolic levels.

Fatty Liver

Fatty liver is very common with Type 2 diabetes. The liver is the body's distribution center for fat. When performing normally, it not only creates fat, but exports it to other areas of the body. When fat is released from the body's tissues, the liver safely removes it from the blood. Disruption of this function of the liver results in its inability to dispose of fat in a healthy manner so fat cells accumulate and take up residence in this organ instead. This can eventually lead to cirrhosis, liver failure, and/or liver cancer.

When I was first diagnosed with diabetes, I also learned I had developed fatty liver. Over time, I was healed from this by taking milk thistle and other herbs that cleansed and healed my liver. See the supplementation section for more information.

Neuropathy

The nerves in your body have a coating called a "myelin sheath". This protective layer of the nerve is similar to that of a cable with the plastic coating outside that protects the internal wiring. High levels of glucose in the blood destroy the myelin sheath, exposing the nerve and this is what causes the tingling and numbness in neuropathy. If neuropathy isn't managed, it can result in the inability to move your legs or arms and also may create ulcers on the skin which won't heal even with antibiotics, possibly even resulting in amputation of a limb.

I want to pause here to tell you about my personal experience with neuropathy. My situation was extremely severe and truly frightening. However, if you're suffering from this yourself, or if you have a loved one going through it, please know that *it can be reversed*. It won't happen overnight, but if you take the Nerve Support Formula Vitamin B12 supplement *at large doses every day*, your body will heal. I found this product online made by Realhealthproducts.com. Your doctor may suggest getting a Vitamin B12 injection every few weeks but that did not work for me. I only felt better the next two days but after that time, my neuropathy worsened.

Currently, the drugs prescribed by doctors for treating the symptoms of neuropathy will not heal the body - they merely mask the pain and numbness *(and sometimes have terrible side effects that only compound the problem)*. As mentioned before, some medications for neuropathy can lead to suicidal thoughts.

The first time I had diabetes, I had severe numbness and tingling in my arms, legs, and feet. My legs and feet were even turning purple, and I could barely walk and had extremely low energy. Imagine waking up each morning and wondering if you're going to be able to move your legs and get out of bed. As time went on, the neuropathy I was experiencing got to the point where I could barely walk up the stairs.

I tried several brands of B12 from various manufacturers but none of them worked. I tried taking them when I ran out of the Nerve Support Formula but they didn't work. Only massive doses of Vitamin B12 can heal neuropathy, and in my experience Real-healthproducts.com provides the best quality. Their version of B12 contains methylcobalamin, which regenerates and heals nerve cells over time. Their supplements are created in "food form" which the body recognizes as food and is therefore well absorbed and utilized by the body. I experienced no negative side effects at all while taking this supplement and whenever I took the pills, within 20 minutes I could feel the nerves in my hands and feet tingling.

Gradually over time, my legs started to become stronger, my arms tingled less and the numbness decreased. My legs were still a light purple when I stood up and I still experienced some small degree of the symptoms, but it wasn't so bad that I couldn't walk anymore. After eight months my body had healed itself completely from all neuropathy. This was due to keeping my blood sugar under 100 every day, eating healthy, taking the proper supplements, and exercising with weights, walking, and jogging.

Years later, the second time my blood sugar rose, I had a completely different set of symptoms. My new symptoms included stomach pain, ringing in the ears, and dizziness whenever I stood up - almost fainting on a number of occasions. Since these symptoms were different from what I experienced the first time, I didn't recognize it for what it was and I was really desperate for answers, going to several different doctors to learn what was wrong. Unfortunately, none of these medical professionals figured it out either. I even went to a gastroenterologist who examined me and was unable to find anything wrong. I then had a CT scan of my abdomen to determine if there were any problems with my internal organs and/or stomach, but it too came up with negative results.

After my second experience with new symptoms of neuropathy and weight gain (of about 25 lbs), I realized I had stopped taking all of my supplements when I moved into a new home and that this caused my blood sugar levels to spike again. I was so focused on the move and setting up all my belongings, I forgot to take my vitamins and supplements. Several months went by and my blood sugar began to rise. After about six months I started becoming dizzy and when I stood up I felt like I was going to faint. I had chronic ringing in my ears, I was exhausted all the time, and had a hard time making it through the day. My A1C had risen from 5.1 to 6.3 in about 9 months and I rapidly regained the weight I'd lost.

It wasn't until I searched on the internet for neuropathy symptoms that I discovered that the new symptoms I was suffering from were also signs of neuropathy and an indication that the diabetes had indeed returned. Once I had this knowledge, I knew how to handle it. I began taking a large daily dose of the Nerve Support supplement. The neuropathy gradually went away again in approximately four months.

As I followed this regimen, the nerves in my brain healed first, decreasing the lightheadedness and dizziness I'd been feeling whenever I stood up. Next, the pain in my stomach went away, and finally, the ringing in my ears came to an end. During all this time, I also continued my diet and exercise program, lowering my blood sugar fro 6.3 to 4.8.

It's important to note that B12 alone is not enough to heal the damage that's been done to your nerves. If you do not also implement and follow a strict diet and exercise program, your blood sugar will continue to be high and continue to damage the protective sheath around your nerves. You will need to combine the diet and exercise program in this book in order to heal completely.

Additionally, many chemotherapy patients have taken the Nerve Support Formula and were healed from their neuropathy. Neuropathy can be caused by many medications and treatments for cancer.

Porter Ranch Gas Leak

As if I hadn't had enough neuropathy in one lifetime, I was exposed to a large amount of chemicals from the Aliso Canyon gas leak in November 2015 in Southern California. After being endangered by the methane gas and other toxins coming from the leaking well, I began to have symptoms just as I had during my first case of neuropathy. I experienced severe dizziness, ringing in my ears, inability to stand or walk, and feeling weak and tired. I didn't have tingling or numbness in my limbs because this was a different form of neuropathy.

Since I knew what was happening to me, I knew what I needed to take to heal. Again, I began taking massive doses of the B12 supplement and after about 3-4 months, my body healed again.

On a side note, if you have pets that are suffering from neuropathy, this same treatment will work for them as well (although in much smaller doses).

Chapter Four

Causes Of Type 2 Diabetes

Although genetics may play a role in causing Type 2 diabetes, it's clear that there is a direct correlation between poor diet and lack of exercise as originating factors in people who get the disease. This situation tends to increase as we age. However, even if your diabetes has a genetic link, repeated studies have proven that it doesn't matter. By eating right and exercising, *you can turn off the gene expression.* This means that through discipline and good habits, you can prevent type 2 diabetes from happening even if it runs in your family. This is an extremely important fact to mention. As mentioned earlier, my family had no history of diabetes yet I developed it anyway. Many people who have a history of it in their families don't get it in life if they live a healthy lifestyle, so gene expression is not considered a deciding factor in getting diabetes.

Poor Diet

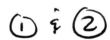

The only things you should be thinking about when you're about to eat, are "how will this food bring nutrition and energy to my body?" and "will it heal me or protect me from disease?" Once these questions become part of your decision-making process, your life will change forever. You should be eating to live, not to feed your depression, anxiety, guilt, shame, or some other emotion. If you're an emotional eater, I highly recommend looking for a therapist who specializes in eating disorders because if you don't fix this problem now, there's no point in continuing this program. You need to get to the root cause of the disorder or you may never stop the self-destructive behavior. Ultimately, this may even solve other issues of which you're not even aware (see the alternative treatment in chapter 8 for the name of my therapist).

Harmful foods

The main offending culprits in obtaining Type 2 Diabetes are sugars and high glycemic carbohydrates. Here's a rough breakdown of the foods that are harmful and why they should be avoided:

Sugars and Carbohydrates

Obviously it's not a good idea to consume sweets in the form of cookies, cakes, doughnuts, and sodas, but you may not be aware of some of the hidden forms of sugar that are also contributing factors in diabetes. Unfortunately, these are present in foods that appear to be good for us in the form of "bad carbohydrates", or carbohydrates that break down into sugars quickly and get into the bloodstream, causing a spike in blood pressure and blood sugar. Potatoes, white rice, pasta, and breads with white flour (bagels, buns, pizza dough, donuts, etc) are all examples of high glycemic carbohydrates. Fruit juices often contain heavy amounts of sugar.

High Fructose Corn Syrup

If you're diabetic, pre-diabetic, or just want to know the one food ingredient to avoid at all costs, it is high fructose corn syrup (HFCS). This is a sweetener made from corn starch that has been processed by glucose isomerase to convert some of its glucose into fructose. It's an ingredient found in many things (many of them hidden) such as ketchup, frozen foods, fruit yogurt, syrups, desserts, baked goods, sodas, fruit drinks, and other condiments. It causes your blood sugar to spike and can damage your liver. The sugars are extracted through a chemical enzymatic process resulting in a chemical and biological compound commonly known as high fructose corn syrup. As use of HFCS has increased, so have levels of obesity and other health related problems. Almost all nutritionists agree that HFCS consumption is a major culprit in the nation's obesity crisis.

The prevailing theory states that the body processes the fructose in high fructose corn syrup differently than it does cane or beet sugar, which in turn alters the way metabolic regulating hormones function. It also forces the liver to push fat into the bloodstream. The end result is that our bodies are essentially tricked into wanting to eat more and at the same time, we are storing more fat.

A single 12 ounce can of soda can have as much as 13 teaspoons of sugar and some of that sugar can be in the form of high fructose corn syrup.

Large doses of high fructose corn syrup have been proven to literally create holes in the intestinal lining allowing damaging byproducts of toxic bacteria and partially digested food proteins to enter your blood stream and trigger the inflammation which is at the root of obesity, diabetes, cancer, heart disease, dementia, and accelerated aging.

Milk and cream

Milk and cream also contain lactose, which quickly converts into blood sugar and this is why they're considered a high glycemic carbohydrate. Unsweetened almond milk is a healthy substitute and can even be used as an ingredient when milk is used in a recipe, or when you need some cream for your coffee. If you really need a sweetener, you can add a few drops of Stevia. Stevia is a natural sweetener found in a plant and has been used for centuries in Asia and other parts of the world.

Glycemic Index

Foods are categorized according to the Glycemic Index (or GI), which ranks them with numerical values in order of how quickly they're metabolized into glucose. Those foods with a high GI, such as refined carbohydrates and sugars, are rapidly turned into glucose, driving up blood sugar levels quickly.

The Glycemic Load Index is based on the same concept as the GI, but takes into account the quality and quantity of food. This is determined by the GI of a food plus the amount of available carbohydrates (excluding fiber) in a standard serving. For example, a large carrot and a cup of spaghetti have similar GIs, yet the carrot contains only 5g of available carbohydrates while the spaghetti contains 38g, giving them GL's of 2 and 16, respectively. Therefore, they have dramatically different effects on blood sugar.

Foods with a low glycemic index value like vegetables, beans, and some fruits cause a slow, sustained level of release of glucose into the bloodstream. They'll keep both your blood sugar and insulin levels from spiking and provide a steady source of energy.

Carrots, watermelon, pineapple, and other fruits with a high GI were once thought to be bad for diabetics, but are now considered to be acceptable.

Saturated fats and trans fats

Bad fats, like trans fats and saturated fats, can increase cholesterol and lead to heart disease. The worst offenders of saturated fat are bacon and sausage, ground meat, dairy products like cream, cheese, butter, milk, sour cream, and processed foods. Trans fat is also usually found in processed foods like bakery items, chips, crackers, cereals, french fries, and fast foods.

Your best bet in avoiding unhealthy foods is to stay away from things that are already prepared like TV dinners, fast foods, and snacks because they often contain these harmful ingredients and more. Such packaged foods are created with the idea of making you addicted to them. The better they taste, the more you'll want them. Quite often, they even include chemicals that can make you addicted to their food. Many of these chemicals can be detrimental to the body. For instance, artificial sweeteners may seem like a good alternative to real sugar, but sometimes they still contribute to diabetes. Use Stevia sweetener whenever possible.

To be safe, try to prepare your own meals using mainly vegetables, fish, poultry, herbs, spices, and healthy fats like avocados and olive oils. A word of caution though - if the diet you provide for your children is too strict and completely deprives them of the things other children get to enjoy, they may overindulge in junk food as adults.

Eating healthy

Eating healthy is not more expensive than fast food, and in most cases it is actually cheaper. Believe me, if you don't eat right, the costs of numerous doctor visits, medical expenses, prescription drugs and surgery will be far more expensive and time consuming. For instance, my business was put on hold while I recovered. This is an unaccounted for expense as there's no way I can calculate the earnings I lost during that time frame, but I have no doubt it was a lot. And it's not just a financial price we pay when we don't take care of our health. Many of the medications used to treat diabetes and related symptoms can create other health problems and cause even more damage to our bodies, such as elevating liver enzymes or other negative side effects, which can disrupt life. In some cases, the price we pay is the pain during and after surgery - like amputation, or a kidney transplant.

On that note, keep in mind that the food industry invests a lot of money in research to find out which ingredients and tactics make humans more addicted to their food and commercials in order to sell their products to you. I've even seen some commercials where they use a model in a bikini to advertise a hamburger. This is an all-time low. In psychology, it's known as a "trigger", which can be an image or word that evokes a feeling associated with a desire. In the case of the model eating a greasy, fattening hamburger, you'll think of her every time you eat one, and when you think of her, you'll want a burger (even if it all just takes place at the subconscious level). This is a really deceptive practice in our society that has far reaching effects on the health of our population. Do not fall for this game. They don't really have your best interests in mind - they only care about making profits and if it means tempting you with models in bikinis to make their stock price go up, they'll continue making these types of commercials. Another example of this shady tactic is product placement. Companies pay big money to have their items placed in the best locations in stores to entice you into purchasing them on impulse. Pay attention to this the next time you're at the store. You'll see gum, candy, and other junk food right next to you in line at check out.

Lack of exercise

These days our society is largely characterized by a sedentary lifestyle. Many of us drive to and from work and sit in offices all day. By the time we get home from work, few people have any energy left to even consider working out or cooking and end up eating fast food instead.

I've tested my blood sugar after eating healthy meals and it would not go lower until I started exercising. After that, it really began to drop. This is due in part to the fact that muscle burns blood sugar day and night, even when you sleep, so strength training in particular is highly beneficial. If you don't maintain an exercise program in addition to a healthy diet, your blood sugar may remain high.

Exercise helps lower blood sugar, regulate levels of cholesterol and triglycerides, decreases the risk of heart disease, removes toxins from your body, and reduces the fat content of the liver. Not to mention that a regular exercise program helps you lose weight, have more energy, and feel better about yourself. After you start getting into shape you'll realize how much more energy you will have. Also your appearance will change and you'll gain more confidence and be more conscious of your decisions on what you should and shouldn't eat.

Psychological reasons for overeating

I have to admit I was an overeater due to depression from a bad breakup. I did not feel happy at the time and indulged in too much processed food. I didn't even realize how I was destroying my body because of my depression. Looking back, I should have seen a psychologist to help me deal with my emotions, but instead I turned towards food to make me feel better. I know that a lot of people overeat because they're unhappy about something. I strongly suggest you find a good therapist to address your depression rather than turning towards food to feel better. Chances are the issue can be understood in a different way and healing can begin before you destroy your body with processed, fatty, sugary food.

In fact, I had to undergo Eye Movement Desensitization Reprogramming (EMDR) in order to finish this book because every time I started to work on it, I would remember all the events from the experience and have to stop working (see the "alternative resources" section in chapter 8 for more information).

Chapter Five

Diet and Micronutrients

Although things like cancer, strokes, and heart attacks seem to appear suddenly, the truth is, they actually build up over time due to an accumulation of bad lifestyle choices, stress, and toxins. Since Type 2 Diabetes is a dietary disease, the treatment for it needs to be dietary - and the good news is that food can be used as medicine. There's a tremendous amount of nutritional science that shows that certain foods can actually heal your body and reverse pre-cancerous cells and other ailments, prevent illnesses, and maintain ideal health.

For the most part, the key to eating right is to prepare and cook your own food but unfortunately, I know that isn't always possible for most of us due to our busy lifestyles so when your time is limited, a lot of supermarkets offer fresh, healthy options that are already prepared for you. A normal portion size of animal protein is about the size of the palm of your hand.

Every few days I go to Whole Foods market and buy prepared foods such as salmon, chicken breasts, or turkey in sizes that are already cooked and seasoned, as well as the perfect portion of protein for me. I then reheat the food in my microwave over the next few days. By having food readily available to reheat, I've been able to prevent overeating.

I always have a large salad at least once a day using a variety of vegetables. Many vegetables contain enzymes, which only can be released when you're chewing them. These enzymes are extremely important in providing your body the nutrients that you can't get from a multivitamin or mineral pill alone.

One way to avoid eating fast food or binge eating at restaurants is to keep snacks like cashews, almonds, bananas, and apples with you at all times. They're full of fiber and keep you full for hours.

Portion sizes

When you go to a restaurant, chances are you'll be given a meal that is twice or three times the amount of food needed. In fact, in most cases that one meal is enough calories (or more) than your entire daily needs. In most cases, the *appetizers* at restaurants are the actual portion size of the meal you should be eating. The restaurants do this to make more money from each individual diner. Think about it. If they only served portion sizes that we should eat instead of what we are given, then they would only make around half the amount of money per person. In addition, the amount of carbohydrates, starches, sugars, and anything else they use in their sauces and food make the meals unhealthy for everyone. In most cases, you should only eat half of your meal at the restaurant and get the other half to go.

The government website - diabetes.gov - sells trays which have the correct portion sizes for meals and lists what to eat (high glycemic carbohydrates vs. low glycemic carbohydrates) and what not to eat. If you're struggling with portion size, it might be worth it to invest in a tray to help you eat the right amounts of food to maintain optimal health.

It is also worth mentioning that the high levels of sugar in popular coffee drinks have as many calories as a regular meal (and in some cases more). They're loaded with sugar, cream and many other high glycemic ingredients as well as caffeine (which spikes your heart rate as well as blood sugar). These are to be avoided at all costs.

My diet for the first six months

For the first six months, this is what I ate every day with only small variations:

✳ Breakfast:

Regular oatmeal warmed with hot water, cinnamon, blueberries, strawberries, blackberries, and raspberries. Oatmeal is full of fiber and keeps you full for hours. It also lowers cholesterol. The berries have antioxidants and other minerals which the body needs.

Black coffee (with no cream or sugar added). For sweetener, I added 4-5 drops of Stevia liquid to the coffee, which was more than enough to make the coffee taste good enough.

There are some studies which support that consuming cinnamon lowers blood sugar, but there have been other studies that showed it did nothing, so the debate on cinnamon continues.

✱ Lunch and/or dinner:

I usually ate chicken breast, turkey, or salmon with a large salad made up of ingredients like kale, spinach, arugula, red onions, mushrooms, broccoli, cauliflower, carrots, tomatoes, and kidney beans.

Salad dressing: Balsamic vinegar, Red Wine Vinegar, or Apple Cider Vinegar and flax oil with lignans and omega-3 oils.

The ingredients of the salads I ate every day are:

- Kale and spinach
- Red onions
- Broccoli
- Olives
- Peas
- Mushrooms
- Cauliflower
- Carrot
- Celery
- Radish

 beets

✱ Snacks I ate everyday

A handful of almonds, cashews or walnuts a few times a day.

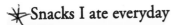

Drinks:

I only drank water and as much as I wanted during meals. I didn't drink any fruit juices, soda, or sweetened or diet drinks of any kind during this entire time.

It is also important to mention that you should remove the skin from all the chicken you eat because the skin contains the most amount of fats. When I ate chicken, I either bought it skinless or removed the skin myself.

My thoughts on eating sweets and desserts

If you do happen to eat junk food or overeat a sugary meal, make up for it by running a few extra miles or training longer the next time you exercise. However, if you really want to lose weight quickly, go cold turkey and don't eat any junk food at all.

I want to point out that after I fully recovered, I was able to eat desserts such as ice cream, cake, frozen yogurt, and chocolate every day in small portions. Eating at the diet I listed above is not realistic and could lead to binge eating (meaning you don't eat bad food for a period of time and then all of a sudden go crazy and eat them until you can't eat anymore). This is not healthy. It is better to treat yourself to something every day (especially on days you exercise). That is the only way you can maintain this lifestyle.

Fasting (D@5-7pm) (B@7am)

Another important method I used was fasting (even though I didn't realize it at the time). I wouldn't eat breakfast on most days that I ate a late dinner. By not eating for 12-14 hours, my insulin levels dropped along with my blood sugar and my body burned the food in my digestive tract at a slow steady rate throughout the night and mornings.

Fasting is a dietary method that Dr. Fung heavily advocates for bringing down insulin levels. He says that when you're not eating, your insulin levels naturally drop on their own accord, breaking the cycle of chasing after rising levels. As you practice fasting over time, you won't become insulin resistant and you'll lose weight more easily.

Micronutrients in foods

When I created my own diet, I instinctively knew that salads were beneficial to me. I wasn't sure why but after I came across Dr. Joel Fuhrman's video on *"Immunity Solution"* and I realized why the salads were healing my body and helping me lose weight. Somehow, deep down inside I knew that eating spinach, kale, cabbage, carrots, red onions, mushrooms, tomatoes, cauliflower, and olives along with a small portion of animal protein would help me regain my health.

Dr. Fuhrman suggests going on a diet that's primarily vegetarian, but several doctors I spoke to suggested eating small portions of animal protein due to the amino acids and other nutrients you can't get from vegetables.

According to Dr. Fuhrman, when you treat diabetes with insulin, it causes weight gain and that it is a fat storage hormone and it builds up in the belly and it requires blood vessels to feed it nutrients. Many nutritional science studies were done to prove that a normal immune system was related to healthy foods. He suggests eating a high micronutrient diet consisting of mostly vegetables and fruits.

In a recent scientific study (2012), the results of the study demonstrate that 90 percent of type 2 diabetics reverse their diabetes within six months on a Nutritarian diet. After 7 months on the high nutrient density diet, the mean A1c dropped from 8.2% to 5.8%, with 62% of participants reaching normal A1c normal levels of less than 6%. In addition, there was a substantial reduction in blood pressure and triglycerides.

The direct link to this study can be found here:

https://www.drfuhrman.com/content-image.ashx? id=65m12xy24xsjpvi3uuoa7e

This study shows that diets low in animal protein and fiber and micronutrients improved glucose tolerance and overall glycemic control as well as decreased insulin resistance. The diet consisted of micronutrients (phytochemicals and antioxidants) from greens, fruits, nuts and seeds and beans. This high nutrient density diet was designed to reduce cravings and overeating and on lowering oxidative stress.

Dr. Fuhrman's entire book *Eat to Live* is based on his research regarding a diet that's mostly plant based. He states that many phytochemicals are released into the mouth by chewing vegetables and which actually heal the body, protect against disease, slow the aging process, and help you lose weight.

He discovered the following foods contain the highest micronu-trients: *Ms Dash*

- Kale
- Collard greens
- Bok choy
- Mushrooms
- Tomatoes
- Strawberries
- Onions
- Flax seeds

Dr. Fuhrman also came up with an acronym to describe these foods to eat on a daily basis to maintain your health and lose weight. It is known as "**GBOMBS**".

Here are the foods contained in GBOMBS:

- Greens – Kale, spinach, arugula,
- Beans – kidney and black beans *(low-sodium) rinsed*
- Onions – red onions
- Mushrooms – any kind of mushroom
- Berries – blackberries, blue berries, raspberry's
- Seeds – walnuts, almonds, cashews, etc

These particular green vegetables contain compounds called Isothiocyanates (ITC's). The ITC's are released when you chew, chop, or blend vegetables. The cell wall releases an enzyme called myrosinase that forms when you chew and are released into the body. There are over 120 types of ITCs and most of them remove carcinogens. Juicing or blending fruits and vegetables has the same effect as chewing them releasing the enzymes. These vegetables also fill your stomach and make you feel full as they are slowly digested into the blood stream. They are all low glycemic so you can eat as much of them as you want.

Beans

Beans have resistant starch that is a carbohydrate that doesn't get absorbed quickly into the digestive tract and works its way into the colon and gets broken down by bacteria.

You'll lose weight from eating beans. They also improve the good bacteria in the stomach and dramatically reduce rates of colon cancer by 50% when they're eaten twice a week. They make you feel full, lose weight, and protect you from cancer.

(low- sodium)

Onions

Studies have shown that onions cause a 50-80% reduction in cancer. Organosulfide compounds are released when you chew on them just like when you cut open an onion and it causes your eyes to tear up. The same chemical reaction happens in your body which is very beneficial at removing carcinogens. Tomatoes are very beneficial for preventing cancer. There have been hundreds of studies showing the benefits from eating tomatoes.

Mushrooms

Mushrooms are the greatest food at preventing cancer. It is best to consume at least 2-5 grams of them a week.

Mushrooms contain the following:

- Antigen binding lectins – they stick to surfaces of abnormal cells so the body can remove them
- Antiogenesis inhibitors – they inhibit enzymes which restrict oxygen and nutrients to abnormal cells. Fat secretes hormones and require blood vessels to feed it nutrients. Mushrooms stop this from happening.
- Aromatase inhibitors – These prevent the body from making excess estrogen. They also protect against breast cancer

Berries have a low glycemic index meaning they get digested slowly and the carbohydrates are minimal. They protect against dementia and cancer. In numerous studies strawberries have been proven to reverse cancer. Seeds and lignens derived from seeds – Flax seeds reduced breast cancer cells when consumed. Less than 1 milligram a day of lignens reduced breast cancer by 70%.

Cholesterol removing foods

Plant sterols, also known as phytosterols (the plant's cholesterol), are naturally occurring substances that are found in fruit, vegetables, beans, whole-grain products and most vegetable oils.

When you eat plants with phytosterols, they fill up the cholesterol receptors in the intestines and as a result, allow bad cholesterol to be flushed out of the body. Experts recommend that to get the maximum cholesterol-lowering benefits, you should be getting between 1,500 to 3,000 milligrams of plant sterols per day through your diet and/or supplementation. To begin to see any benefits you need to get a minimum of 800 milligrams of phytosterols per day.

Foods to avoid due to their high glycemic load:

- White potato
- White rice
- Pasta made from white flour
- Cake or ice cream
- Corn
- Sweet potato
- Grapes
- Rolled oats
- Whole wheat
- Mango

Foods to eat which have a low glycemic index:

- Lentils
- Apples
- Kiwi
- Green peas
- Squash
- Kidney beans
- Black beans
- Watermelon

- Oranges
- Cashews
- Strawberries

These foods are great sources of carbohydrates with a low glycemic load and are high in fiber and micronutrients.

TOXIC HUNGER
Anabolic / Catabolic curve

Dr. Fuhrman created the term "toxic hunger" to describe the difference between true hunger and hunger based eat processed foods. He describes two phases that the body goes through after eating food - the "anabolic phase" and the "catabolic phase".

Anabolic phase – The anabolic phase is when you're eating and digesting. It is referred to as the building phase where you are consumed food.

Catabolic phase – The catabolic phase is when your body is breaking down the food to turn it into energy.

According to Dr. Fuhrman, during the anabolic phase your glucose rises in a process similar to *filling* up the gas tank of your car. The catabolic phase is analagous to driving your car and *using* the gas that you filled it up with. Your body repairs itself and circulates toxins. When you eat processed foods, the toxins and free radicals build up which make people uncomfortable and they get withdrawal symptoms such as headache and growling stomach so they eat more to make themselves feel better. If you eat again it stops the catabolic phase and you feel better because you go back into the anabolic phase. That's *toxic hunger*. The American diet is so toxic people become addicted to food and instead of feeling true hunger, they eat when they are uncomfortable and return to the anabolic phase.

You want to remain in the catabolic phase as long as possible and only eat when you have true hunger after 4-6 hours. It is always better to remain in the catabolic phase until you become truly hungry. After your last meal of the day, it is always best to not eat until the morning and possibly skip breakfast. This is the intermittent fasting I mentioned earlier.

True hunger is felt in the mouth and throat. Your body won't be hungry if you eat high volume*s of salads or* foods with lots of micronutrients. You can eat as much of these foods as you want and never have to worry about diets again. This is due to the fact that your body senses that the food has all the nutrients in it that you need and therefore, you won't get hungry for longer periods of time.

The reason diets don't work is because you can't ignore your body's nagging drive to eat. The body doesn't feel well because its always requiring nutrients.

Chapter Six

Supplements

Supplementation is a big part of keeping your blood sugar low. Alpha Lipoic Acid, chromium, vanadium and gymnema are extremely important supplements that keep your blood sugar low. Below are some of the supplements I took during my six month period of healing (and continue to take). You can buy most of the vitamins and minerals separately but I prefer to take a supplement that contains most or all of the ingredients I need. It is much easier to take and also more cost effective.

The following supplements lower blood sugar:

- Glucose Support Formula (from Realhealthproducts.com) – (contains a combination of the vitamins and minerals listed below)
- Chromium - this mineral metabolizes glucose
- Vanadium - glucose and cholesterol control
- Gymnema Sylvestre - stabilizes blood sugar and controls weight
- White Kidney Bean Extract - prevents starch from converting into glucose
- Green coffee bean extract - controls blood sugar and suppresses appetite and increases metabolism

- Garcinia Cambogia – lowers blood sugar, reduces appetitite, helps you lose weight.
- Apple Cider Vinegar – lowers blood sugar, improves digestion, and improves immunity (along with many other health benefits)
- Alpha Lipoic Acid - good for peripheral neuropathy and lowering blood sugar

The following supplements are good for blood pressure and overall health:

- Hawthorn - lowers blood pressure and treats chronic heart problems
- Calcium - lowers blood pressure
- Magnesium - lowers blood pressure
- Potassium - lowers blood pressure
- Fish Oil - lowers your triglycerides and cholesterol and is good for your heart and brain
- Vitamin D – lowers blood sugar and may reduce obesity
- Milk Thistle - lowers blood sugar, decreases fatty liver, and inflammation
- CoQ10 – contains an enyme which is good for your heart
- Multivitamin – beneficial for overall health

How They Work
Glucose Support Formula (from Realhealthproducts.com)

This supplement contains a combination of vitamins and minerals found in the listed in the previous page. This is an "all in one pill" and is very effective at lowering and maintaining a normal blood sugar level. This supplement uses "food form" technology, which means it's easily absorbed by the body since the body recognizes it as food.

Chromium

Chromium is essential to proper metabolism and maintaining safe sugar levels. Excess insulin depletes your body's chromium that is critical to blood sugar metabolism. As a diabetic, you're most likely deficient in this nutrient. If you ever wondered where your "sweet tooth" and sugar cravings come from, it's most likely due to chromium deficiency. Calcium and Magnesium are also depleted by excess insulin, which can cause many problems as they are critical to over 200 biochemical processes in your body.

If you are insulin resistant, these important nutrients may causes you to be deficient in other vitamins and minerals as well, including zinc, selenium, vitamin E, vitamin C, vanadium, B Complex vitamins, essential fatty acids and many more.

Vanadium

Vanadium is a trace mineral found in a wide variety of foods. Research suggests that vanadium supports normal blood sugar levels and insulin activity in the body and also promotes and supports healthy cholesterol levels.

Gymnema Sylvestre

Gymnema Sylvestre is an Ayurvedic herb that's been used in India for over 2,000 years, since the 6th century BC, to support healthy and normal blood sugar levels in the body.

As soon as I eliminated carbohydrates and started taking vanadium, chromium and gymnema, fish oil, I began to lose weight at a very rapid pace (almost 2 pounds a day for the first 5 months). My blood sugar went down from a fasting blood sugar reading of 115 average to about 96 and I started feeling better and having more energy. I no longer felt sluggish and could easily make it through the day. The dizziness and fainting almost went away, although taking the Nerve Support Formula during this time helped heal my body while I kept the blood sugar levels down.

White Kidney Bean Extract

Supplements containing extracts made from white kidney bean are used for weight loss because they are thought to act as "starch blockers" by inhibiting the starch-digesting enzyme amylase which turns the starch you eat into absorbable sugar. Several studies have been performed showing that taking this supplement promotes weight loss when taken concurrently with meals containing carbohydrates.

Garcinia Cambogia

Garcinia cambogia is a citrus fruit that grows in Southeast Asia. It is an extract from the fruit's rind, hydroxycitric acid (HCA), which has been used for cooking, but it has also been used for weight loss. HCA works by making you feel full, reducing your appetite, and affecting your metabolism. This has led many to believe it works as a natural weight loss supplement. There have been some studies that prove that this supplement can influence fat metabolism. Several studies have found that both mice and humans experience an increase in fat metabolism after taking HCA.

I personally used this for months and definitely noticed a decrease in hunger and maintained a healthy body weight (even without exercising for several weeks at a time). I found myself waiting longer periods of time before becoming hungry.

Green Coffee Bean Extract

The healing properties come from the green coffee bean and is not found in regular brewed coffee or espresso. Raw coffee beans are naturally green (it's the roasting process that gives them their dark color). However, by roasting, the beans lose the chlorogenic acids, which are naturally occurring antioxidants that are key for stimulating weight loss and stabilizing blood sugar. By increasing the efficiency of your body's metabolism through enhancing body temperature, your body's fat burning ability will be increased. This also releases glucose into your bloodstream, which forces the body to turn to fat cells as a source of energy. In doing this, your body uses stored fat for energy and thus, you will experience fat loss.

While this process prevents sugar from circulating in your system and inhibits fat absorption, it's stimulating the liver, encouraging your body's metabolism to work at peak performance.

Green coffee bean extract lowered my blood sugar dramatically, increased my metabolism and weight loss, and it also suppressed my appetite.

Apple Cider Vinegar

Research shows apple cider vinegar (ACV) taken daily can help prevent blood sugar spikes because it helps with starch and carbohydrate absorption. Nutritionists and doctors agree that reducing the glycemic response in the body is especially important if you're diabetic or have insulin resistance, but anyone can benefit. Ingesting ACV with a higher carbohydrate meal can decrease post-meal blood glucose levels.

Vinegar has been shown to have numerous benefits for insulin function and blood sugar levels:

- Improves insulin sensitivity during a high carbohydrate meal by 19-34% and significantly lowers blood sugar and insulin responses
- Reduces blood sugar by 34% when eating 50 grams of white bread
- 2 tablespoons of apple cider vinegar before bedtime can reduce fasting blood sugars by 4%

ACV also can help you lose weight (especially around the waist). A study of obese individuals showed that daily vinegar consumption led to reduced belly fat, waist circumference, and lower triglycerides. Studies have also shown that vinegar lowers blood pressure and also contains chlorogenic acid which has been shown to prevent LDL cholesterol from becoming oxidized, an important step in heart disease.

ACV also kills many types of bacteria and pathogens. It has traditionally been used for cleaning and disinfecting. Studies show that ACV inhibits bacteria from growing in food. However, make sure to talk to your doctor before taking this vinegar so your blood sugar doesn't go too low.

I experimented with my body many times to test the efficacy of Apple Cider Vinegar on my blood sugar levels. I noticed that when I used it, my blood sugar dropped at least 20 points within an hour and kept it low.

The normal dose of ACV is a tablespoon before meals. You can find great recipes to make it easier to drink online. Adding honey will make it more bearable to drink. I normally drink 2-3 tablespoons every day diluted with water. Organic, unfiltered apple cider vinegar (like Bragg's) also contains "the mother", strands of enzymes and friendly bacteria that give the product a murky appearance.

Alpha Lipoic Acid

Alpha Lipoic Acid (ALA) is used for improving peripheral neuropathy and helps control glucose levels. ALA also helps to detoxify the liver of pollutants, blocks cataract formation, and reduces blood cholesterol levels. In addition to all of this, it also protects the mitochondria in our DNA from free radicals. It slows the aging process and decreases the risk of cancer, autoimmune diseases, cardiovascular disease, and brain dysfunctions. Everyone should be taking it, but depending upon how high your glucose levels are, you'll probably need to take between 600 mgs and 1200 mgs per day.

ALA is one of the most potent antioxidant vitamins known. Of all the major antioxidants, only ALA has the ability to work in both water soluble and fat soluble environments in the body. Being able to penetrate cellular membranes throughout the body also means that ALA can cross the blood-brain barrier to exert its protective effects against neurological diseases, such as Alzheimer's disease.

Numerous studies have shown that ALA improves glucose tolerance as well as the nerve complications associated with full-blown diabetes. ALA is similar to insulin because it increases glucose uptake in insulin-resistant cells.

European researchers treated 12 overweight adults suffering from Type 2 diabetes and were given 600 mg twice daily over a period of four weeks. They found that ALA treatment increased peripheral insulin sensitivity in patients with Type 2 diabetes in just four weeks.

Lipoic acid also shows great benefits in overcoming neuropathy once diabetes has taken hold. A number of clinical studies have demonstrated its effectiveness in diabetic neuropathy. Many researchers believe this may be due to its strong antioxidant power in improving the damaged nerves. One study involving 328 diabetic patients with peripheral nerve problems revealed that a 600 mg daily intravenous treatment of ALA is safe and effective for overcoming characteristic symptoms such as pain, burning, and itching in the feet after just three weeks of treatment.

Supplements which lower blood pressure and are beneficial to overall health

As mentioned above, Calcium, magnesium, hawthorn, and potassium are all instrumental in controlling blood pressure. All four of these ingredients work naturally with no side effects and in many cases, are better than blood pressure medicine. I had really bad side effects from several different medications prescribed by my doctor. The important thing to remember is make sure to talk to your doctor and monitor your blood pressure while weaning off prescription drugs for hypertension. You don't want to stop taking your medication suddenly, because the supplements may not work for you, or you may need to adjust your dosage gradually (increasing or decreasing it until you find the right amount which maintains your blood pressure in a normal range). If you take too much hawthorn, calcium and/or magnesium and drink apple cider vinegar, they may lower your blood pressure too much. If you take too little, it may go too high. This is why it's important start gradually and monitor it daily with a blood pressure monitor and work with your physician to monitor it. Wait and see how your body responds to the supplements and then slowly increase the dosage of the supplements and lower the drug until you can eventually get off the medication.

Hawthorn

Hawthorn comes from a flowering shrub that is part of the rose family and has been used for centuries to lower blood pressure and treat chronic heart problems for decades. It has been used for diseases of the heart and blood vessels such as congestive heart failure, chest pain, and irregular heartbeat. It is also used to treat both low blood pressure and high blood pressure, hardening of the arteries, and high cholesterol.

Calcium

Calcium is important for the creation of teeth and bones, but it also contributes to the health of many other systems, including the muscular, circulatory and nervous systems.

Dairy products are rich in calcium, as are some nuts and leafy green vegetables. According to the Linus Pauling Institute, adults need between 1,000 and 1,200 milligrams of calcium per day.

Magnesium

Magnesium benefits several metabolic functions. It helps your body use protein, produce energy, and adjust blood pressure levels. The standard doses are between 310 and 420 milligrams of magnesium daily.

Potassium

Potassium helps with nerve health, helping to conduct electric impulses that allow your muscles to contract and your heart to beat properly. Both males and females need 2,000 milligrams of potassium per day from the time they turn 10 years old.

Calcium, magnesium, and potassium taken together in one pill is much more effective at lowering blood pressure since they work synergistically together

Fish Oil

Fish oil has a number of benefits to the body. First, it lowers triglycerides, a common problem with diabetics.

Omega-3 fish oil contains both docosahexaenoic acid (DHA) and eicosapentaenoic acid (EPA). Omega-3 fatty acids are essential nutrients that are important in preventing and managing heart disease.

Findings show omega-3 fatty acids may help to:

- Lower blood pressure
- Reduce triglycerides
- Slow the development of plaque in the arteries
- Reduce the chance of abnormal heart rhythm
- Reduces the likelihood of heart attack and stroke
- Lessen the chance of sudden cardiac death in people with heart disease

The American Heart Association recommends that everyone eat fish at least twice a week. Salmon, mackerel, herring, sardines, lake trout, and tuna are especially high in omega 3 fatty acids. If you have heart disease or high triglyceride levels, you may need even more omega 3 fatty acids.

If you have high triglycerides you should take up to 6 pills a day (a daily dose of 10800 mgs of fish oil) and at the very least, two tablets per day. I took the highest dose to lower my triglycerides from 495 to 185 in 6 months.

Fish oil drastically lowered my triglyceride levels into the normal range in just a few months. See the lab section for more information.

Vitamin D

Vitamin D is important for the regulation of calcium and phosphorus absorption, maintenance of healthy bones and teeth, and helps prevent against multiple diseases and conditions such as cancer, multiple sclerosis, and Type 1 diabetes.

Vitamin D has multiple roles in the body:

- Maintains the health of bones and teeth
- Supports the health of the immune system, brain, and nervous system
- Regulates insulin levels
- Supports lung function and cardiovascular health

Vitamin D is produced when sunlight converts cholesterol on the skin into vitamin D3. The metabolism of vitamin D may be affected by some medications, including statin drugs. Another interesting fact is that vitamin D deficiency has been seen in up to 80% of hip fracture patients.

Milk Thistle Extract

Milk thistle is from a plant. It comes in capsule or liquid form. The liquid form is much stronger and faster in aiding the body than pill form since the liquid goes into the blood stream faster because it bypasses the digestive system. Regular pills have to be digested and diluted in the stomach and liver first.

Several years ago, I had to take strong antibiotics for 4-6 weeks. I felt some pain and tenderness in my liver area and had blood tests to confirm the liver enzymes were elevated and it was strained. I took several capsules of milk thistle and several droppers of the liquid form every day and I began feeling better within hours of taking one dropper full of the extract. After a few weeks, the pain in my liver area was gone and my blood test results showed my liver enzymes were back in normal ranges.

Taking milk thistle helped me have more energy, clearer skin, lose weight, and sleep better. Today, most people take one or more prescription drug, but these can seriously affect your liver function. A lot of older folks take 5 or more drugs. Together, they can really cause harm to your liver and slow its function - even if you don't drink.

The liver needs to be protected since it's responsible for a large percentage of your immune functioning and also stores glycogen and cleanses your blood. In order for your immune system to fight off disease, it's important to keep your liver in the best possible condition. Milk thistle is almost the only substance that can improve liver function. It can also lower cholesterol and blood sugar, works as an antioxidant and fights inflammation. Some people have even claimed it relieved them of their arthritis. In addition to its primary function of supporting liver health, milk thistle has shown to be helpful in lowering blood sugar and LDL, as well as helping with insulin resistance.

There are additional supplements that help heal the liver and detoxify it. A few examples of these herbs are dandelion, artichoke, beets, grape seed extract, L-glutathione, L-carnitine, cape bush, chicory, yarrow and black nightshade. You can buy an all in one supplement containing most or some of these ingredients at any health food store or online.

COQ10

Coenzyme Q10 (COQ10) supports the heart. As we age, production of this enzyme diminishes. It is a substance similar to a vitamin. It is found in every cell of the body. Your body makes CoQ10 and your cells use it to produce the energy your body needs for cell growth and maintenance. It also functions as an antioxidant that protects the body from damage caused by harmful molecules. Coenzymes help enzymes with digestion of food and perform other processes, and they help protect heart and skeletal muscles.

Many claims are made about CoQ10. It's said to help prevent heart failure, as well as cancer, muscular dystrophy, and periodontal disease. It's also said to boost energy and speed recovery from exercise. Some people take it to help reduce the effects certain medicines can have on the heart, muscles, and other organs.

Chapter Seven

Exercise

In order to completely reverse Type 2 Diabetes and lose weight, you will need to change your diet *and* follow an exercise program. There is no exception to this, even if you can only walk for 15 minutes a day. Exercise makes insulin work more efficiently in the body and lowers blood sugar, and resistance training is the most effective form of exercise you can do. If you are too sick to exercise, you should at least change your diet and take supplements until you are strong enough to walk. If you can walk without any problems, then you should walk at a normal pace for at least 30 – 60 minutes a day. You burn just as many calories walking as you do running. When traveling throughout Europe several years ago, I lost more weight walking around sightseeing than I did during my regular staggered workouts.

The key to maintaining exercise is to find a sport or activity that you enjoy. It can be anything such as dancing, basketball, tennis, swimming, hiking, biking, etc. If you enjoy the activity, chances are you will continue to do it and over time it will help you get into shape.

Over the years, I have tested my blood sugar using the glucose monitoring kit hundreds of times, experimenting with different exercises to determine which one worked better. I did this to understand the condition so I could control it. I would perform the blood test before each exercise and immediately afterwards to see which exercise reduced my blood sugar the most. After years of experimentation, I have found that weight training combined with high intensity interval training (HIIT) is by far the most effective way to lower your blood sugar and to *keep it low because muscle burns glucose 24 hours a day.* The next best exercise is jogging and/or running followed by walking for at least 30 minutes a day. The more you weight train, the lower your blood sugar will be. Ideally, the best workout routine is jogging or running for 30 minutes followed by weight training. You can lift weights before running but it is better to warm up the body by jogging for at least ten minutes.

The workout program I demonstrate in this book is something I have used for the past 20 years and continue to use to this day. Whenever I have a setback or something happens in life where I can't work out every day, I have to start over using these exact methods mentioned here.

The description of my workout routine is described in this chapter, but it is always better to learn to lift weights by watching a video than by reading a book. I provided it just for illustration purposes, but the ideal way to learn how to train with weights is by watching the workout video found on Endingdiabetes.net. This training program is for beginners. If you are a professional athlete, pro bodybuilder, or have trained for years with weights, then you will not find this section as useful as the diet or supplementation sections.

I wanted to emphasize how important it is to give yourself enough time between workouts so your muscles can heal. I've split up the workout routine so you are working out every other day and working different muscle groups of your body on different training days. For example, on Monday you can train chest and back, Wednesday you train legs, Friday you train shoulders and arms.

I designed this workout routine so your body will become equally proportioned, hitting every major muscle group at least once a week. This will give you an even and well-balanced aesthetic physical appearance and allow your muscles to recover from workouts between days by splitting up the workouts.

It is always a good idea to stretch the muscle groups you plan on working out before, during, and after your routine.

You will also need to increase your protein intake daily by eating more chicken, fish, turkey, and occasionally, some beef. I prefer to use a whey protein shake combined with egg whites. You can also buy liquid egg whites online.

You actually build muscle after you work out. During exercise, you are tearing the fast twitch fibers in your muscle. Fast twitch fibers are the muscle fibers which fatigue rapidly during exercise. They rebuild faster than long twitch fibers. They also use large reserves of glycogen rather than oxygen rich blood for quick energy. Slow twitch fibers are smaller and take about three times longer to contract after receiving stimulus. These muscles are needed for posture and movement and in the back and leg muscles.

What causes soreness the next day or longer is the breakdown of the fast twitch fibers and possibly slow twitch fibers depending on how long you've worked out for. Afterwards your body begins to heal itself by rebuilding the muscle fibers. This continues for several days until the muscle has recovered. The more you train, the more you'll build more muscle over time as you continue to tear and rebuild the micro fibers in your muscles.

Benefits of exercise and weight training

- Builds lean muscle which in turn promotes fat loss and increased metabolism
- Lowers blood pressure
- Gives you more energy, alertness, and strength
- Improved sleep quality – you will sleep better, fall asleep faster, and wake up refreshed
- Glucose will remain low as muscle burns glucose day and night
- Increases libido
- Enhances your mood
- You'll become more confident, stronger, and positive psychologically

Endingdiabetes.net has a video that you can buy to watch repeatedly so you can really understand the information demonstrated in this section. Other workout videos don't include useful and realistic information on diet and supplementation and certainly nothing about reversing diabetes or weight training for beginners. All of these topics are covered in greater detail on my site.

My video is about realistic ways to stay in shape, with a simple diet to follow. It's designed for beginners—for someone who has never worked out a day in their life, someone who's rebounding from an illness, or for someone who just wants to learn how to maintain a healthy and manageable exercise and diet plan. I've used this plan repeatedly for the majority of my life and it has always worked for me. Whenever I had a setback, I'd always resort to this program to rebuild my muscles.

If you've had a break in your workout routine it is very important to start with light weights again to rebuild the fast twitch muscle fibers. I've seen numerous serious injuries from people who started training where they had left off when they last trained. Even just a few weeks of time between workouts will require you to start at a lower weight.

If you can master the weight training aspect of this program, you'll be able to add more weight to each set as you continue to build muscle from working out. Eventually, you'll move on the intermediate and advanced levels. As you build muscle and get into shape, you'll gain more confidence in your appearance, which will motivate you to continue training harder and longer even more.

Things To Consider

- A great way to jumpstart your exercise program is to hire a personal trainer. I hired one to help me get back into the routine and practice the proper weight training form for lifting weights so I wouldn't injure myself. Another advantage to hiring a trainer is that paying an hourly fee in advance will definitely keep you motivated to train or you will lose out on your deposit.
- Walking burns as many calories as running or jogging, but running speeds up your metabolism more and will make you burn fat faster.
- The key to exercising is consistency, even if only a few weeks at a time.
- If you work out really hard one day, get enough rest to recover. Listen to your body and don't overdo your workouts.

You need time to recover, even from light workouts. You need to build up the muscle fibers first to gain strength to do the hardcore workouts later on.

- Listen to your body and if you're feeling deeply fatigued from travel, work, or lack of sleep, you shouldn't work out. Give your body the rest it needs so you can exercise again the following day.
- The first 20-30 minutes of your workout can be difficult, but once you get past that point, you'll get a second wind and have more energy than ever before due to endorphins and adrenaline.
- Your heart is a muscle. If you over train in the beginning of your workout program, you could have a heart attack. At the very least, you can strain your muscles so much that lactic acid will build up rapidly, causing your muscles to feel pain and burning. You'll be so sore the next few days you won't ever want to work out again.
- What you do for a living makes a huge difference in how many calories you burn and what your caloric needs will be. For example, someone who works in construction needs a lot more calories than an office worker who sits at a desk all day.
- It is critical to train with weights if you have diabetes. Weightlifting builds muscle and muscle uses blood sugar for energy.
- Get a deep tissue massage every few weeks, as it does wonders for the body.

The key to this training program is that it is designed for working people, students, or anyone whose busy lives prevents them from working out every day. This is a common sense basic routine that will allow you to get all the training you need in one hour or more.

In the beginning, I believe it is more important to work out every other day - not every single day. You need to take a day off in between workouts to recover as you progress through this program (however, if you have the energy to train on consecutive days and aren't sore, then work out as often as you like). This is important not only physically but also psychologically. If you train every day, your muscles will not have enough time to recover and you'll be sore. Even though some sources say you can exercise during muscular pain, I highly advise against it because you could injure yourself. More importantly, forcing yourself to work through it creates more pain, and could make you completely lose interest in weight training and exercise.

If you are sore from the prior day's workout, you'll be miserable during the following day and your mind will link pain with exercise and that's the last thing you want to happen. You need to ease into your routine with baby steps, working your way up gradually and slowly, listening to your body along the way, and when you feel you can go longer, faster and harder, you can train harder, longer, and with heavier weights.

There are other reasons not to over train in the beginning as well. First of all, you need to get into a habit of exercising, and they say it takes 3 weeks for a routine to become a habit. Second, once the habit forms, the process becomes easier and you'll actually begin to look forward to it. You want exercise to be a pleasurable experience. Go at your own pace.

If you decide to hire a personal trainer or exercise with a friend, they may inadvertently try to push you to train harder with the intention of helping you, but they may actually be risking an injury.

Sometimes people mean well when they say, "Come on, one more rep" or "Keep up with my pace", or they may try to motivate you by adding more weight, but in reality your body is different from theirs, and it's not worth tearing a muscle or ligament just to impress them. This could cause so much pain that you can barely move the next day or even be out of commission for months and have to start all over again. It's better to go at a slow, steady pace building upon your earlier workouts than suffer a setback.

Setbacks are part of life. I've had so many over the years that I could write a book on them. If you get sick, travel for work, or have something in life interfere with your training program, you need to ease your way back into training. The longer you've taken time off, the slower you need to start again and the lighter the weights need to be. I've had to revert back to this beginner's style of training over and over again after setbacks kept me from training consistently.

The Workout Routine

As I mentioned earlier, it is nearly impossible to learn how to lift weights properly by reading a book. I have only listed the workout routine for illustration purposes. Please see the "Weight Training for Beginners" video listed on the site, endingdiabetes.net for a more complete, thorough demonstration on how to exercise.

We'll start by exercising all of your major muscle groups using basic core weight training techniques. Train with weights every other day and most importantly, do your lifting in this order:

- Chest and Back
- Legs
- Shoulders and Arms

You can alternate this routine to whatever you are most comfortable with, but I believe that alternating days for your muscle groups is better because when you lift weights with your upper body you're using secondary muscles. For example, when you work out your chest muscles, you are also using your triceps as secondary muscles. When you're working out your back you're also using your biceps. So by breaking up your workouts in this way you're giving the secondary muscle groups in your upper body time to recover in between workouts.

When I first began exercising, the only exercise I could do is walk. I walked 20-30 minutes a day and then gradually worked up to an hour. Over time, I began to add weight training to my workouts and saw a dramatic difference in weight loss, energy, glucose levels and overall feeling of well-being.

Body part exercises:

Chest

- Flat bench presses
- Inclined bench press
- Dumbbell lifts

Back

- Lat Pull downs
- Rowing
- Dumbbell lifts

Biceps

- Barbell curls
- Dumbbell curls
- Isolation curl using machine

Shoulders

- Shoulder press (front, back and center)
- Dumbbell lifts

Triceps

- Cable pull downs
- Dumbbells

Legs

- Squats (show leg distance and angle of feet pointed forward)
- Leg Presses
- Calves
- Hamstrings
- Lunges

Stomach

- Sit ups (regular and to train the oblique muscles)
- Crunch machine

This entire workout should take you no longer than 60-90 minutes.

You should have a high protein meal or protein shake within 45 minutes after your workout. This is so the protein will start rebuilding the muscle. There are many brands of protein shakes but the fastest absorbing protein is whey.

Chapter Eight

Alternative Resources for treatment

Over time, I found some great resources that helped me reverse this disease and return to optimal health. I discovered **Whitaker Wellness Institute in Newport Beach, California**. I received LED light treatments, which enhanced the healing of my neuropathy symptoms in my legs and arms, IV treatment to lower my blood pressure, hyperbaric oxygen therapy to increase the concentration of oxygen levels in the organs and tissues of my body, and supplements to lower my glucose and blood pressure levels. The LED light treatments are used to treat burn victims and speed up the healing in tissues in the body.

Under the care of **Dr. Andre Berger at Rejuvalife.com**, I received a combination of medication and supplements, as well as weight loss management treatment. Dr. Berger performed comprehensive tests (both physical and mental) before assessing a plan of treatment. He even sent me to a sleep center for the insomnia I was experiencing at the time. At Dr. Berger's facility, he conducted Body Mass Index tests, which measured the body fat percentages, lean muscle, and much more (see lab section for more information). He also requested Glucose Tolerance Tests, cortisol and thyroid blood tests to get an overall picture of my health and to assess a treatment plan.

Whitaker Wellness Center – www.drwhitaker.com Address: 4321 Birch St, Newport Beach, CA 92660. Phone: 949-851-1550

Whitaker wellness is an alternative treatment facility that treats diabetes on many levels. They have a group of doctors who are specialized in treating diabetics and have many forms of treatments such as LED light therapy (which helps heal the nerves from neuropathy and can prevent amputations), a diet and lifestyle program, oxygen chambers to increase oxygen in the body (great for people who have had recent strokes), acupuncture, and intravenous treatments to help heal the body. They also have their own supplement store which carries many of the supplements I mentioned in this book.

Dr. Whitaker's philosophy and treatment protocols involve a combination of therapeutic lifestyle changes, vitamins and other targeted nutritional supplements, as well as additional natural therapies that work in tandem to jumpstart the body's innate healing ability. He believes that with the right guidance, education, and therapies, we are all capable of achieving optimal health and well-being, and that no patient is too sick to improve his or her health. This, he says, is the true meaning of "health care"— achieving wellness, not managing disease.

Dr. Andre Berger - 9400 Brighton Way #405, Beverly Hills, CA 90210. Phone: (310) 276-4494

Dr. Andre Berger at www.rejuvalife.com is an all-encompassing doctor who treats patients with a multi-pronged approach that includes both supplements and pharmaceutical medications to help patients. He provides a psychological questionnaire to determine if your body needs specific nutrients along with numerous blood tests, Body Mass Index tests to determine lean muscle mass, body fat percentage and other measurements.

Dr. Jason Fung – www.intensivedietarymanagement.com

Dr. Fung is a Canadian nephrologist. He's an expert on intermittent fasting and treatment for people with Type 2 diabetes. His facility also treats patients without the use of insulin or other common diabetic drugs. You can see his YouTube videos at

https://www.youtube.com/user/drjasonfung

Dr. Joel Fuhrman – www.drfuhrman.com

Dr. Fuhrman, author of the books *Eat to Live* and *The End of Heart Disease* and *The End of Diabetes*, is a board certified physician with over 25 years of practicing nutritional medicine. Both of his books give very careful instructions on how to remove diabetes medications and reverse diabetes for both the physician and lay person with hundreds of scientific references. He has created an eating plan which helps individuals improve their immune system, lose weight, lower blood pressure and blood sugar, and provides them with all the nutrients to live healthy lives. Dr. Fuhrman created the term "Nutritarian" to describe a diet that is nutrient-dense and plant-rich, and includes anti-cancer super foods, which also facilitate weight loss. These foods supply both the right amount of macronutrients (protein, fat, and carbohydrates) and the vital micronutrients (vitamins, phytochemicals, and minerals) that unleash the body's incredible power to heal itself and slow the aging process, giving the body renewed vitality. Dr. Fuhrman gives personalized guidance to hundreds of patients through his website Dr-Fuhrman.com and has a member center to assure optimal results and prevent the confusion and misinformation that abounds on this subject.

Dawn Zeinert - http://www.dawnzienert.com Address: 11712 Moorpark St #111, Studio City, CA 91604. Phone: (323) 413-7456

Dawn Zeinert helped me recover from trauma in many areas of life – stress, anxiety, depression, hostile work environment, bad breakups and much more. She is experienced in working with survivors of trauma, including Adult Children of Alcoholics (ACOA), and victims of sexual, physical, and emotional abuse. She's trained and experienced in EMDR therapy (explained in great detail in the psychological section). In addition, she has extensive experience in working with couples who are experiencing relational conflict. She provides you with the tools you need in order to help you heal.

Eye Movement Desensitization and Reprocessing (EMDR)

Eye Movement Desensitization and Reprocessing (EMDR) is a therapy technique that is well researched and proven effective for the treatment of trauma. Therapists and scientists don't really understand how EMDR works in the brain. However, they do know that when a person is really distressed their brain can't process information as well as it usually does. One moment becomes "frozen in time," and remembering a trauma may feel as if you're still experiencing it for the first time because the images, sounds, smells, and feelings haven't changed. Such memories have a lasting negative effect that may interfere with a person's behavior and mood.

Eye movement desensitization and reprocessing seems to have a positive effect on the way that the brain processes information. After successful EMDR treatment, you'll no longer relive the images, sounds, and feelings when the event is recalled. You'll still remember what happened, but the emotional response to the memory is lessened or even gone completely.

EMDR works by putting the brain in a "dream state" that's identical to rapid eye movement during sleep. The brain is then allowed to process the memories. After 4 sessions of this treatment, I was able to continue writing this book without any disturbing emotions from my experience.

EMDR is very useful for the following conditions:

- Panic attacks and phobias
- Grief and disturbing memories
- Pain disorders
- Eating disorders and body image problems
- Performance anxiety and stress reduction
- Addictions
- Sexual and/or physical abuse
- Stress and anxiety issues often respond well to EMDR
- Difficulty trusting others

- Being attracted to people who just aren't good for you
- Feeling guilty without knowing why
- A history of being physically or emotionally abused as a child
- Self-blame, self-consciousness, shame, or guilt
- Chronic or excessive anger and sadness
- Worry, anxiety, and obsessive thinking
- Unpleasant feelings and mood swings
- Negativity, pessimism, and irritability

To learn about the development and history of EMDR see www.emdr.com and emdria.org.

Blood Tests

If you don't have health insurance, you can get lab tests from www.labcorp.com and request the appropriate tests listed in the labs section. You don't need a doctor's order to get these done. The Complete Blood Count (CBC) with lipid panel checks a wide variety of issues in your body. It tests the liver function, kidneys, red blood cell count, white blood cells, glucose, cholesterol and triglycerides and much more (see the first lab test in the labs section to see which one I'm referring to).

You can always add additional items to get tested as well, such as the Hemoglobin A1C test and other markers which are not included in the CBC. For example, one test for men is the Prostate Specific Antigen (PSA) test which measures the amount of prostate specific antigen in your blood.

If you are diagnosed with diabetes, you can request the Glucose Tolerance Test (a sample of mine is in the lab section). This is the test which measures your blood sugar every 2 hours after drinking a sugary drink which the lab provides. This test checks for insulin resistance and determines whether or not your body ability utilizes sugar.

If you don't have health insurance

If you don't have health insurance, a great resource to choose from a variety of plans is www.ehealthinsurance.com. I've personally used this company to buy my own insurance since I'm self employed, and there are many low cost plans to have just in case of an emergency. With the our health care laws in flux, this information is subject to change.

Chapter Nine

Antibiotics and Pro-Biotics

Antibiotics

Antibiotics are great at killing bad bacteria in your body due to infections. However, the negative side of taking them is it also kills off all your good bacteria in your stomach. The good bacteria in your stomach actually makes up a big percentage of your immune system. If you take a lot of antibiotics, your good bacteria will be diminished and your white blood cell count may become too low, as did mine. My white blood cell count dropped to levels lower than normal after completing two rounds of antibiotics.

In order to rebuild both your good bacteria and your immune system, you should take probiotics to maintain healthy levels of helpful bacteria in your gut (ideally during or after your cycle of antibiotics).

After I continued to have sinus problems due to allergies, I took an antibiotic for several months that caused me to have pain in my lower abdomen for almost 6 months. I went to a gastroenterologist who ran all kinds of tests on me just to find out everything was normal. The only thing that healed me was taking probiotics.

Probiotics

The best probiotic I took is a brand called "Bio K Plus", which can be found in health food stores such as Whole Foods and also online. Bio K Plus contains the kind of bacteria found in your gut, replenishing all of the good bacteria that restores immune function and also aids in digestion. Other useful probiotiocs also consist of several billion cultures. Kefir probiotic smoothies and/or regular yogurt contain good bacteria but aren't as strong as Bio K Plus yogurt.

Bio K Plus is used by doctors in hospitals and has the same types of good bacteria found in the human stomach. You can drink a bottle a day or half a bottle, depending on how long you've been on antibiotics. This will keep everything balanced, rebuild the good bacteria in your stomach, maintain and rebuild your immune system, and keep your white blood cell count high. Depending on how long you've been on antibiotics, you will need to use the probiotics for at least a few weeks or longer. If you don't have any symptoms such as abdominal pain, or gas, that is usually a sign you can discontinue probiotics.

Chapter Ten

Blood test results

In this section I will show you proof of how I lowered my blood sugar from 6.8 to 4.8 in less than 6 months and lost 41 pounds. I will also show you the Body Mass Index (BMI) measurements taken during this time and my weight loss and lean muscle mass gains. I have also provided "before" and "after" pictures which show how I changed in appearance.

The first lab shown below illustrates the moment I initially learned something was wrong with my body and requested to have a Complete Blood Count (CBC) performed so I can find out what was happening to me. It shows that my glucose level was slightly out of range, but most importantly I want to show you how out of range the cholesterol and triglyceride levels were.

On page 2, you'll see the triglycerides were 651 and the normal range was 10-160. This is over 5 times the normal range. My cholesterol was slightly out of range but the VLDL was 130 with a normal range of 0-40. These were the first clues that I had diabetes because most people who have it have an elevated fasting glucose level, high cholesterol, and triglycerides.

The following lab tests show the gradual decrease in cholesterol, triglycerides, and A1c levels.

MetroLab, Inc.

16550 Ventura Blvd. #402, Encino, CA 91436
tel. (818) 724-4300 e-mail: metrolabinc@aol.com fax: (818) 728-4384

RESULT REPORT

Behrouz Dardashti, M.D.
Pathologist, Medical Director

4-7-10

INSTITUTION
Josephson, William M.D. Y.
17075 DEVONSHIRE ST. SUITE 100
NORTHRIDGE, CA 91325
TEL: (818) 831-7767
Fax: (818) 831-2757

PATIENT
Babayans, Brian
DOB: 2/11/1965   GENDER: M

PATIENT TEL: 818 730-9419

DATE/TIME COLLECTED	DATE RECEIVED	DATE REPORTED
4/07/2010 19:26	4/07/2010	4/13/2010

ACCESSION #: 10040723   REQUISITION #:   CHART #:

STATUS FINAL.
KS:

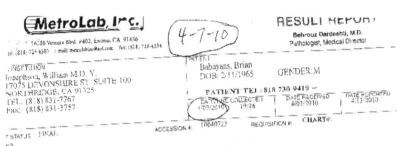

TESTS	RESULTS IN RANGE / OUT OF RANGE		UNITS	REFERENCE RANGE
CHEMISTRY				
GLUCOSE		111 H	mg/dL	70-105
BUN	9		mg/dL	7-25
CREATININE	0.8		mg/dL	0.5-1.5
POTASSIUM	4.2		mEq/L	3.5-5.3
SODIUM	137		mEq/L	136-145
CHLORIDE	100		mEq/L	98-110
CO2	25		mEq/L	20-31
BUN CREA RATIO	11.4		Ratio	5-40
CALCIUM	9.5		mg/dL	8.6-10.2
ALBUMIN	4.4		g/dL	3.5-5.1
TOTAL PROTEIN	7.0		g/dL	6.2-8.3
SGPT (ALT)		91 H	IU/L	9-60
SGOT (AST)	32		IU/L	10-40
ALK PHOSPHATASE	114		U/L	40-115
TOTAL BILIRUBIN	0.5		mg/dL	0.0-1.2
URIC ACID	6.3		mg/dL	4.0-8.0

LIPID PANEL

CHOLESTEROL — 216 H mg/dL 100-200

(NCEP) NATIONAL CHOLESTEROL EDUCATION PROGRAM GUIDELINES:
  LOW RISK - < 200 MG/DL
  BORDERLINE RISK - 201-239 MG/DL
  HIGH RISK - >240 MG/DL

HDL CHOLESTEROL 28 mg/dL 27-67
  NOTE: MALE   27 TO 68 MG/DL
        FEMALE 29 TO 89 MG/DL

CHOLESTEROL/HDL 7.8 H Ratio 3.6-4.7

LDL (Calculation) 58 mg/dL <100

THE THIRD REPORT (NIH PUBLICATION 01-3670) OF THE NATIONAL
CHOLESTEROL EDUCATION CHOLESTEROL EDUCATION PROGRAM (NCEP)
SUGGEST TREATMENT AND DIAGNOSTIC GUIDELINES BE BASED ON THE
FOLLOWING RANGES FOR LOW-DENSITY LIPOPROTEIN (LDL) CHOLESTEROL:

OPTIMAL TARGET: LESS THAN 100mg/dl
NEAR OPTIMAL/ABOVE OPTIMAL: 100-129 mg/dl
BORDERLINE HIGH: 130-159mg/dl

Page 1

MetroLab, Inc.

16550 Ventura Blvd. #402, Encino, CA 91436
tel (818) 728 4200 e-mail metrolab@hotmail.com fax (818) 728 4204

RESULT REPORT

Behrouz Dardashti, M.D.
Pathologist, Medical Director

INSTITUTION
Josephson, William M.D, Y.
17075 DEVONSHIRE ST. SUITE 100
NORTHRIDGE, CA 91325
TEL: (818) 831-7767
Fax: (818) 831-3757

PATIENT
Babayans, Brian
DOB: 2/11/1965   GENDER: M

PATIENT TEL: 818 730-9419

DATE/TIME COLLECTED	DATE RECEIVED	DATE REPORTED
4/07/2010 19:26	4/07/2010	4/13/2010

ACCESSION # 10040723   REQUISITION #   CHART#:

STATUS FINAL

TESTS	RESULTS IN RANGE / OUT OF RANGE	UNITS	REFERENCE RANGE
HIGH:	100-189 mg/dl		
VERY HIGH:	GREATER THAN 190mg/dl		
VLDL (Calc.)	130 H	mg/dl	0-40
TRIGLYCERIDES	651 H	mg/dL	10-160
HEMATOLOGY			
		10³/uL	4.0-11
WBC	5.8	10⁶/uL	4.7-6.1
RBC	5.66	g/dL	12.0-18.0
HGB	17.4	%	37.0-52.0
HCT	47.5	fL	80.0-99.0
MCV	83.9	pg	27.0-34.0
MCH	30.7	g/dL	32.0-37.0
MCHC	36.6	10³/uL	150-400
PLATELETS	164	%	45-75
GRANULOCYTES %	49	%	15-50.0
LYMPHOCYTES %	35	11 H %	0-10
MONOCYTES %		%	0-7
EOSINOPHILS %	4	%	0-5
BASOPHILS %	1		
SPECIAL CHEMISTRY		%	3.9-6.1
GLYCOHEMOGLOBIN	5.58		
TUMOR MARKERS		ng/mL	0.00-4.00
TPSA	0.67		

Test methodology: ECLIA on Roche Elecsys 2010. Results from different
methods cannot be used interchangeably.

THYROID STUDIES		ug/dL	5.1-14.1
T4	7.0	uIU/mL	0.27-4.20
TSH	<0.01 L	ng/mL	0.8-2.0
T3,TOTAL	1.1		
URINALYSIS			Straw-Yellow
COLOR	Dark Yellow		Clear
CHARACTER	Clear		1.006-1.025
SPECIFIC GRAVITY	1.010		5.0-8.5
PH	7.0	sec	Neg
URINE PROTEIN	Neg	mg/dL	Neg
URINE GLUCOSE	Neg		Neg
URINE KETONES	Neg		Neg
OCCULT BLOOD	Neg		0.2-1
UROBILINOGEN	0.2		

Page 2

If age and sex are not indicated, adult main range is specified.

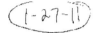

Quest Diagnostics

(1-27-11)

Report Status: Partial

BABAYANS, BRIAN

Patient Information	Specimen Information	Client Information
BABAYANS, BRIAN	Specimen: BN972444F	Client #: 76089294 BH073159
DOB: 02/11/1965 AGE: 45	Requisition: 0000424	BERGER, ANDRE
Gender: M		REJUVALIFE MED ASSOC., INC.
Phone: 818.730.9419	Collected: 01/27/2011 17:22 PST	Attn: ANDRE BERGER, M.D.
Patient ID: 02111965BB	Received: 01/27/2011 22:00 PST	9400 BRIGHTON WAY STE 405
	Reported: 01/28/2011 22:07 PST	BEVERLY HILLS, CA 90210-4711

Test Name	In Range	Out Of Range	Reference Range	Lab
VLDL CHOLESTEROL				
TRIGLYCERIDES	130		<150 mg/dL	EN
VLDL CALCULATION				TH
CHOLESTEROL, VERY LOW				
DENSITY LIPOPROTEIN	27		<30 mg/dL (calc)	
CREATININE, RANDOM URINE	284		20-370 mg/dL	EN
MICROALBUMIN, RANDOM				EN
URINE OX/CREATININE)				
MICROALBUMIN	1.9		mg/dL	
Endnote 1				
MICROALBUMIN/CREATININE				
RATIO, RANDOM URINE	7		<30 mcg/mg creat	

The ADA defines abnormalities in albumin
excretion as follows:

Category   Result (mcg/mg creatinine)

Normal   <30
Microalbuminuria   30-300
Clinical albuminuria > 0R = 300

The ADA recommends that at least two of three
specimens collected within a 3-6 month period be
abnormal before considering a patient to be
within a diagnostic category

LIPOPROTEIN (a)	19		<75 nmol/L	EN
LIPID PANEL				
CHOLESTEROL, TOTAL	197		125-200 mg/dL	EN
HDL CHOLESTEROL		32 L	> OR = 40 mg/dL	EN
TRIGLYCERIDES	136		<150 mg/dL	EN
LDL CHOLESTEROL	138		<130 mg/dL (calc)	EN

Desirable range <100 mg/dL for patients with CAD or
diabetes and <70 mg/dL for diabetic patients with
known heart disease.

CHOL/HDLC RATIO		6.8 H	< OR = 5.0 (calc)	EN
GLUCOSE	97		65-99 mg/dL	EN

Fasting reference interval

SODIUM	138		135-146 mmol/L	EN
POTASSIUM	4.1		3.5-5.3 mmol/L	EN
CHLORIDE	102		98-110 mmol/L	EN
UREA NITROGEN (BUN)	19		7-25 mg/dL	EN
CREATININE W/eGFR				EN
CREATININE	1.09		0.76-1.34 mg/dL	
eGFR NON-AFR. AMERICAN	>59		> OR = 60 mL/min/1.73m2	
eGFR AFRICAN AMERICAN	>59		> OR = 60 mL/min/1.73m2	
CALCIUM	9.5		8.6-10.3 mg/dL	EN
MAGNESIUM	2.3		1.5-2.5 mg/dL	EN
PHOSPHATE (AS PHOSPHORUS)	3.6		2.5-4.5 mg/dL	EN

11022838 - Babayans, Brian   2-28-11

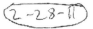
MetroLab, Inc.

16560 Ventura Blvd. Suite 402
Encino, CA 91436
PH: 818-728-4300 FAX: 818-728-4034

Client:
DR. ETEHAD SIAMAK P., M.D.
17075 DEVONSHIRE ST SUITE #100
NORTHRIDGE, CA 91325

Patient Name:
Babayans, Brian
Physician:
Etehad, Siamak M.D.

Patient I.D.	Date of Birth	Age:	Sex:
000098717	2/11/1965	46	M
Accession:	Other ID:		
11022838			

	Date:	Time:	Status:
Collected:	2/28/11	20:06	FINAL
Received:	2/28/11	20:06	
Reported:	3/04/11	13:35	

Test	Normal	Abnormal	Units	Reference
CHEMISTRY				
GLUCOSE	96		mg/dL	70-105
BUN	15		mg/dL	7-25
CREATININE	0.8		mg/dL	0.5-1.3
POTASSIUM	4.3		mEq/L	3.5-5.3
SODIUM	137		mEq/L	136-145
CHLORIDE	100		mEq/L	98-110
CO2	23		mEq/L	20-31
BUN CREA RATIO	19.5		Ratio	3-40
CALCIUM		11.2 H	mg/dL	8.6-10.2
ALBUMIN		5.3 H	g/dL	3.5-5.1
TOTAL PROTEIN	6.9		g/dL	6.2-8.3
SGPT (ALT)		74 H	U/L	9-60
SGOT (AST)	27		U/L	10-40
ALK PHOSPHATASE	102		U/L	40-115
TOTAL BILIRUBIN	0.9		mg/dL	0.0-1.2
URIC ACID	5.2		mg/dL	4.0-8.0

LIPID PANEL

CHOLESTEROL	137		mg/dL	100-200

(NCEP) NATIONAL CHOLESTEROL EDUCATION PROGRAM GUIDELINES:
LOW RISK - < 200 MG/DL
BORDERLINE RISK - 201-239 MG/DL
HIGH RISK - >240 MG/DL

HDL CHOLESTEROL		26 L	mg/dL	27-67

NOTE: MALE - 27 TO 68 MG/DL
FEMALE - 28 TO 89 MG/DL

CHOLESTEROL/HDL		5.4 H	Ratio	3.6-4.7
LDL(Calculation)	75		mg/dL	<100

THE THIRD REPORT (NIH PUBLICATION 01-3670) OF THE NATIONAL
CHOLESTEROL EDUCATION CHOLESTEROL EDUCATION PROGRAM (NCEP)
SUGGEST TREATMENT AND DIAGNOSTIC GUIDELINES BE BASED ON THE
FOLLOWING RANGES FOR LOW-DENSITY LIPOPROTEIN (LDL) CHOLESTEROL:

OPTIMAL TARGET: LESS THAN 100mg/dl
NEAR OPTIMAL/ABOVE OPTIMAL: 100-129 mg/dl
BORDERLINE HIGH: 130-159mg/dl
HIGH: 160-189 mg/dl
VERY HIGH: GREATER THAN 190mg/dl

VLDL (Calc.)	37		mg/dL	0-40
TRIGLYCERIDES		183 H	mg/dL	10-160

HEMATOLOGY

WBC		3.4 L	10^3/uL	4.0-11
RBC	4.83		10^6/uL	4.7-6.1
HGB	15.1		g/dL	12.0-16.0
HCT	42.1		%	37.0-52.0
MCV	87.2		fL	80.0-99.0
MCH	31.3		pg	27.0-34.0

Diagnostics

(4-22-11)

Report Status: Final

BABAYANS, BRIAN

Patient Information	Specimen Information	Client Information
BABAYANS, BRIAN	Specimen: EV9143021	Client #: 93063025 MAIL00
DOB: 02/11/1965 AGE: 46	Requisition: 0005445	WASSER, HARRIS
Gender: M		WASSER MD, HARRIS
Phone: 818.812.9679	Collected: 04/22/2011 14:25 PDT	2950 SYCAMORE DR STE 200
Patient ID: 02111965BB	Received: 04/22/2011 22:58 PDT	SIMI VALLEY, CA 93065-1210
	Reported: 04/26/2011 14:51 PDT	

COMMENTS: FASTING

Test Name	Lo Range	Out Of Range	Reference Range	Lab
LIPID PANEL WITH REFLEX TO DIRECT LDL				
CHOLESTEROL, TOTAL	159		125-200 mg/dL	RN
HDL CHOLESTEROL		17 L	> OR = 40 mg/dL	CN
TRIGLYCERIDES		154 B	<150 mg/dL	UN
LDL CHOLESTEROL	111		<130 mg/dL (calc)	TM

Desirable range <100 mg/dL for patients with CHD or diabetes and <70 mg/dL for diabetic patients with known heart disease.

CHOL/HDLC RATIO		9.4 B	> OR = 5.0 (calc)	LN
COMPREHENSIVE METABOLIC				SN
PANEL W/eGFR				
GLUCOSE	86		65-99 mg/dL	

Fasting reference interval

UREA NITROGEN (BUN)	10		7-25 mg/dL	
CREATININE	0.92		0.78-1.44 mg/dL	
eGFR NON-AFR. AMERICAN	101		> OR = 60 mL/min/1.73m2	
eGFR AFRICAN AMERICAN	119		> OR = 60 mL/min/1.73m2	
BUN/CREATININE RATIO	NOT APPLICABLE		6-22 (calc)	
SODIUM	137		135-146 mmol/L	
POTASSIUM	4.5		3.5-5.3 mmol/L	
CHLORIDE	103		98-110 mmol/L	
CARBON DIOXIDE	26		21-33 mmol/L	
CALCIUM	9.4		8.6-10.2 mg/dL	
PROTEIN, TOTAL	5.6		6.2-8.3 g/dL	
ALBUMIN	4.3		3.6-5.1 g/dL	
GLOBULIN	2.3		2.1-3.7 g/dL (calc)	
ALBUMIN/GLOBULIN RATIO	1.9		1.0-2.1 (calc)	
BILIRUBIN, TOTAL	0.4		0.2-1.2 mg/dL	
ALKALINE PHOSPHATASE		140 B	40-115 U/L	
AST	32		10-40 U/L	
ALT		00 B	9-60 U/L	
HEMOGLOBIN A1c		5.0	<5.7 % of total Hgb	SN

Increased risk of diabetes
<5.7   Decreased risk of diabetes
5.7-6.4   Increased risk of diabetes
6.1-6.4   Higher risk of diabetes
> OR = 6.5 Consistent with diabetes

Standards of Medical Care in Diabetes-2010.
Diabetes Care, 33:Supp 1: S1-S61,2010.

TSH, 3RD GENERATION		<0.01 L	0.40-4.50 mIU/L	SN
T4 (THYROXINE), TOTAL		9 B	4.5-12.0 mcg/dL	RN
T4, FREE			0.8-1.8 ng/dL	
T3, FREE		5 2 B	2.3-4.2 pg/mL	
T3, TOTAL			76-181 ng/dL	
THYROID PEROXIDASE AND THYROGLOBULIN ANTIBODIES				LN
THYROGLOBULIN ANTIBODIES	<20		<20 IU/mL	SN
THYROID PEROXIDASE			<20 IU/mL	SN

COLLECTED: 04/22/2011 14:25 PDT
Printed by Client information on 04/26/11 at 08:01pm

Body Mass Index tests

In this section, I will show you the loss of weight and increase in lean muscle mass in less than 6 months. Below is the general information provided to me from the Body Mass Index results with guidance on amount of calories needed to maintain or lose weight. Dr. Berger began with a 1200 calorie a day limit to help me lose weight.

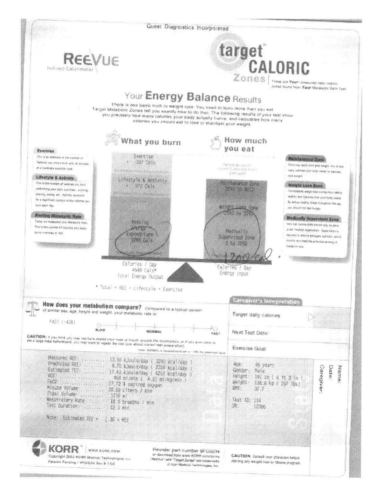

Before my treatment began, my weight was 257 pounds and my body fat percentage was 35%.

InBody — Brian Babayans

REJUVALIFE VITALITY INSTITUTE
9400 BRIGHTON WAY STE 406, BEVERLY HILLS
TEL 310.276.4494

Name(I.D.)	Gender	Age	Height	Date	Time
	Male	45years	6ft. 3. 0in.	11. 23. 2010	14:32:59

Body Composition

Compartments	Values	Total Body Water	Lean Body Mass	Weight
Intracellular Water	77.1 lbs	121.8 lbs	166.5 lbs	257.1 lbs
Extracellular Water	44.7 lbs			
Dry Lean Mass	44.7 lbs			
Body Fat Mass	90.6 lbs			

Body Composition Analysis

		Under	Normal	Over	
Weight				257.1 lbs	
Skeletal Muscle Mass				96.1 lbs	
Body Fat Mass				90.6 lbs	
Intracellular Water				77.1 lbs	
Extracellular Water				44.7 lbs	

Obesity Diagnosis

	Under	Normal	Over
Body Mass Index			32.1
Percent Body Fat			35.2

Segmental Lean Development

	Under	Normal	Over
Right Arm			10.6 lbs
Left Arm			10.2 lbs
Trunk			78.2 lbs
Right Leg			28.5 lbs
Left Leg			28.2 lbs

Body Fat & LBM

Fat Control	- 61.3 lbs
LBM Control	0.0 lbs
Basal Metabolic Rate	2001 kcal

BMI [Body Mass Index] ☐ Normal ☐ Under ☑ Over
PBF [Percent Body Fat] ☐ Normal ☐ Under ☑ Over

Impedance	RA	LA	TR	RL	LL
20kHz	274	292	34.9	242	246
100kHz	242	257	28.4	211	215

Body Composition
Your body is composed of water, dry lean mass (protein and mineral) and fat. Total body water is divided into water inside the cells (Intracellular water) and water outside the cells (Extracellular water). When you are healthy, your body maintains a balanced ratio between Intracellular water (ICW) and Extracellular water (ECW). Keeping these components in appropriate balance is the key to staying fit and healthy. Compositional imbalance in the body is closely related to obesity, malnutrition, edema and osteoporosis.

Body Composition Analysis
Excessive body fat is the cause of many diseases, and it is important to keep your body fat mass in a normal range. Your body fat mass and muscle mass determine your physique. In order to have a firm looking body, it is necessary to have greater muscle mass than body fat mass. An ideal graph would show the SMM to be greater than the body fat mass graph. Extracellular and intracellular water balance is critical for health since the body is composed mostly of water. When extracellular water is abnormally greater than intracellular water for some reason, edema is recognizable.

Obesity Diagnosis
The BMI method is the most common. It evaluates your weight in relationship to your height to assess body fat content. If your BMI is over the normal range, you are considered to be at risk for obesity related diseases. Percent body fat uses a percentage to show how much of your weight is body fat. Percent body fat is able to differentiate between muscle weight and fat weight while BMI does not. BMI is helpful for 'normal' individuals to assess their obesity risk, but percent body fat is based on the composition of the individual rather than solely on their weight. The normal range for PBF is 10~20% for males and 18~28% for females.

Segmental Lean Development
The longer the bar graphs in this section, the better. This section is used to evaluate muscle strength and its distribution throughout the body. The normal or over range represent well developed muscle, while the under range indicates segments of the body that are lacking muscle. When analyzing the results it is helpful to compare the right and left side of the body and the upper to the lower extremities. By comparison you can assess whether your body is balanced or unbalanced.

Body Fat & LBM
Identifies the amount of body fat mass and muscle mass you should gain or lose in order to reach your ideal body composition.
LBM Control • (need more LBM)
0.0 (maintain current LBM)
Fat Control • (need more Body Fat Mass)
- (lose Body Fat Mass)

In this second test taken one month after the last one, you will see I actually gained some weight but my body fat percentage had dropped almost 10%.

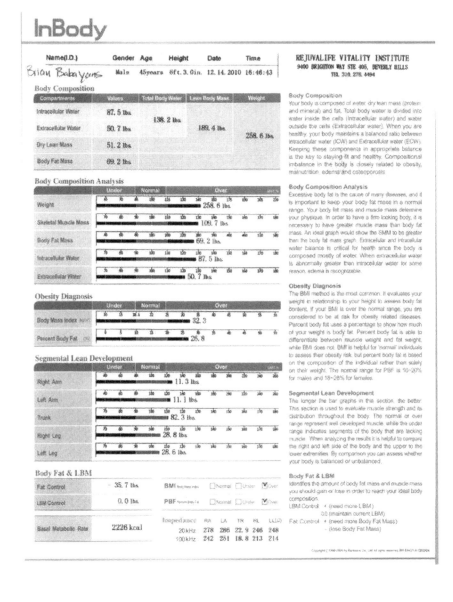

Two weeks later, I dropped another 14 pounds. I also began losing weight in the body fat mass category.

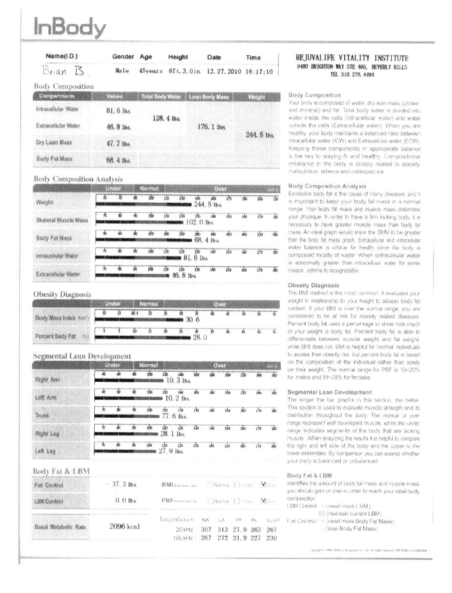

Six weeks later, I lost another 19 pounds from my last test. My body fat mass went from 68 pounds to 52 pounds. My body fat percentage went from 35% to 23%.

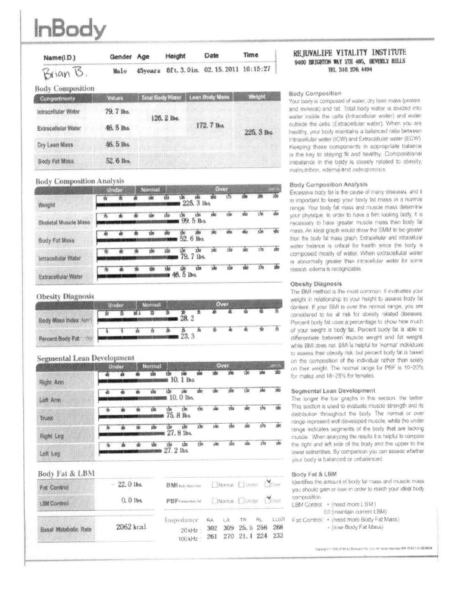

A month later, I lost another 4 pounds, but more importantly my body fat mass went from 68 pounds to 51 pounds.

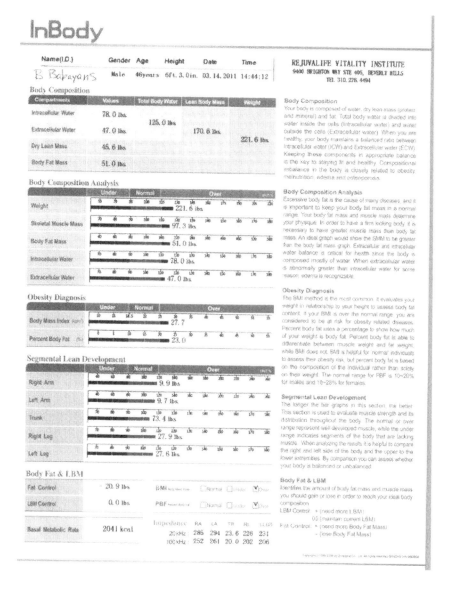

Two weeks later, my body fat mass had dropped to 46% and my body fat percentage went to 20%. Even though I gained a few pounds from the previous test, I began to build lean muscle mass from weight training. You can see the right and left arm increased in weight approximately one pound each.

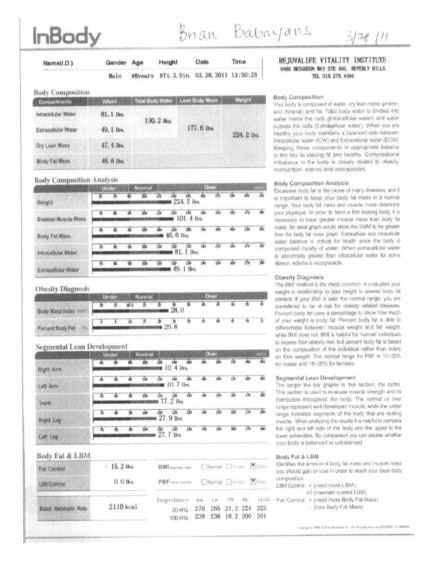

Here is the final test six months from the beginning of my treatment. I lost a total of 17% in body fat, 21 pounds and dropped from 35% body fat to 18% body fat. My lean muscle mass also increased as well and since muscle weighs more than fat, that explains the increase in weight.

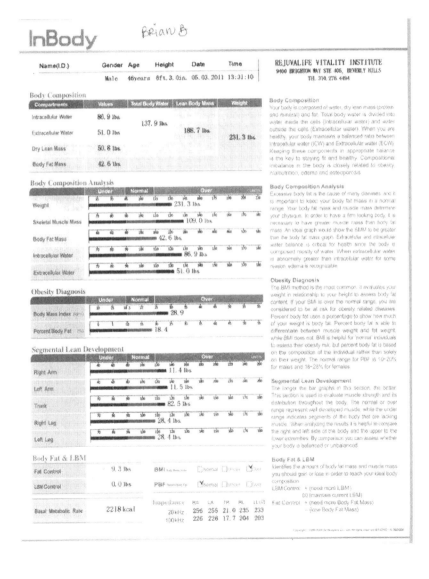

Even though there isn't a final test showing my actual weight loss at the end of 6 months, I weighed myself daily on a weight scale at home and dropped all the way to 211 pounds, a total loss of weight of 41 pounds. But as I began to lift weights on a more consistent basis, my muscle mass grew, and as stated earlier muscle weighs more than fat so my weight actually began to increase even though my fat percentage continued to drop.

Chapter Eleven

Before and After photos

Below are the "before" pictures taken at the beginning of my treatment on Nov, 2011

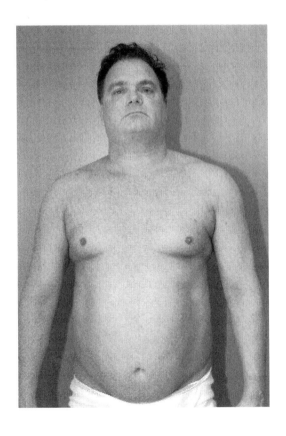

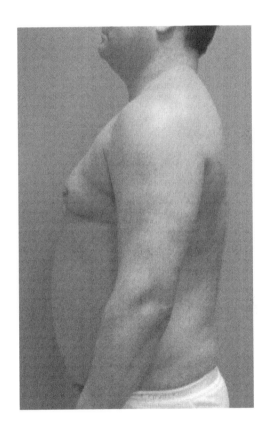

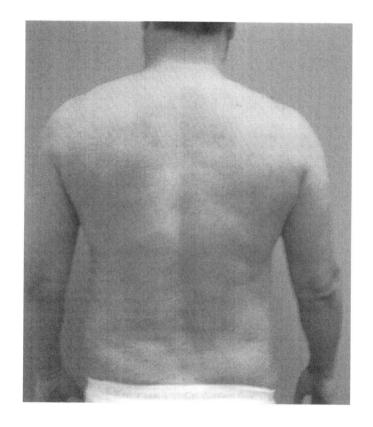

My "after" photos taken 6 months later

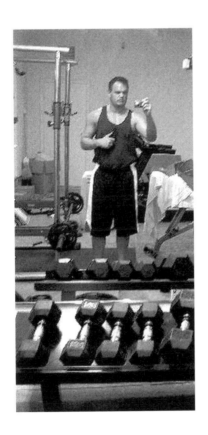

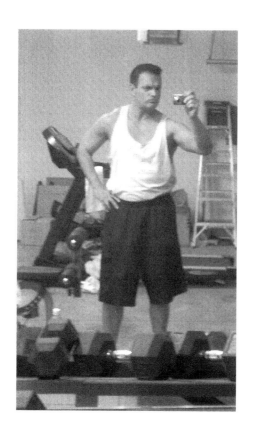

Conclusion

As I have demonstrated through the lab results, body mass index measurements and before and after pictures, Type 2 Diabetes is completely reversible through the diet, exercise and supplementation. I've detailed my entire diet plan for six months going into detail why plant life not only helps you lose weight, but also heal from illness. I created a workout routine that lowers blood sugar quickly and keeps it low. I've listed all the natural supplements that also keep blood sugar low, suppress appetite, restore the PH balance in your stomach, and give your body all the nutrients to heal and thrive. All of these factors combined allowed my body to completely reverse Type 2 Diabetes, heal from severe neuropathy, lose 41 pounds in six months.

I believe that the dangers of modern food are the leading cause of diabetes and also the fact that most people don't know what to eat and are being led into foods that damage their bodies. I strongly urge you to not be seduced by the TV commercials, TV food shows and advertisements that can lead to a life dependent on pharmaceutical drugs and their side effects, decreased health and lifespan and most importantly quality of life.

Regardless of how sick you are from Type 2 Diabetes, I've demonstrated that the body is a natural healing machine, and that you can restore your health. The doctors and facilities I've listed give you an alternative resource to investigate outside of the normal healthcare system.

References

Dunaief DM, Fuhrman J, Dunaief JL, Ying G. Glycemic and cardiovascular parameters improved in Type 2 Diabetes with the high nutrient density (HND) diet. *Open Journal of Preventive Medicine.* 2012 Aug; 2(3):364-371

" Just keep going "
thewalkingmouth . com
veg (raw & cooked)
beans
fruits
raw nuts/seeds
avos
ground flax seeds

salad:

romaine) chopped
arugula)
Mrs Dash - ~~Pestic~~ Fiesta Lime!
califlower rice
pinto beano
mushrooms
onion
walnuts
lo-so salsa

ACV - 2-3T a day (before meals)

Dr. Joel Fuhrman "Eat to Live"
Nutritarian diet

(B) Oatmeal, cinnamon, berries
Black coffee w/ stevia

(L/D) Chicken, Turkey, Salmon
salad

(S) almonds, cashews

Lots of water!
ACV!